W0114459

5-MINUTE CHAIR YOGA
FOR SENIORS

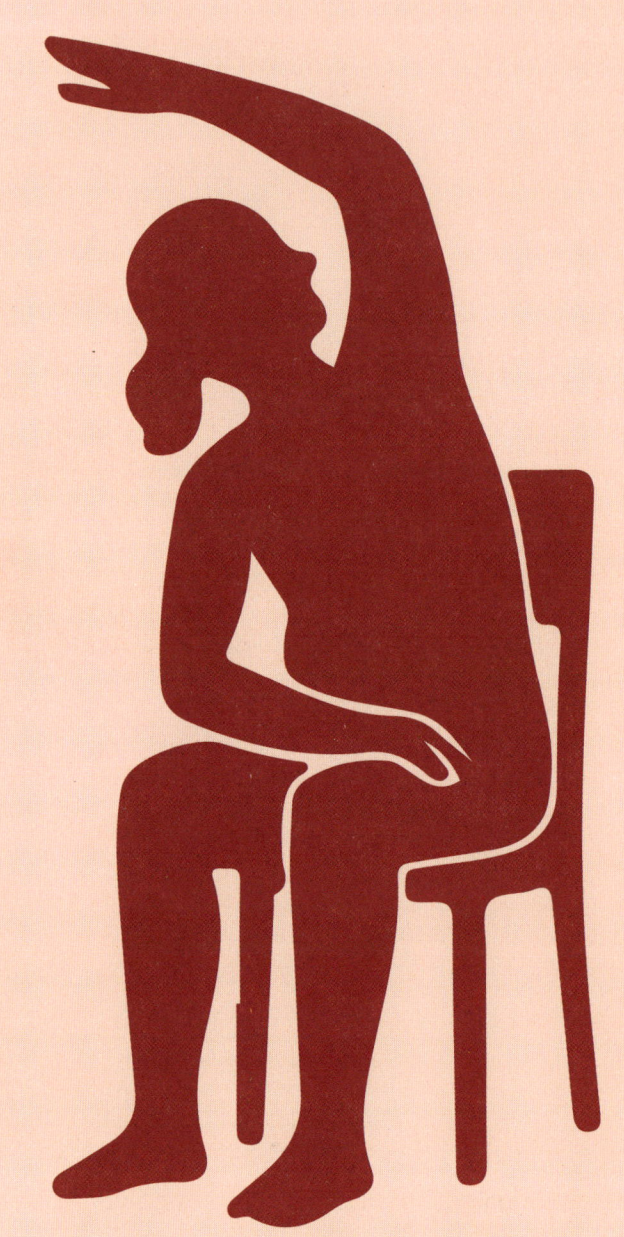

Kierstie Payge Dolezal

5-Minute
CHAIR
YOGA
FOR SENIORS

Simple Exercises to Improve
Mobility and Reclaim Your Confidence

SASQUATCH
BOOKS

Copyright © 2025 by Sasquatch Books

All rights reserved. No portion of this book may be reproduced or utilized in any form, or by any electronic, mechanical, or other means, without the prior written permission of the publisher.

Printed in Colombia

SASQUATCH BOOKS with colophon is a registered trademark of Blue Star Press, LLC

29 28 27 26 25   9 8 7 6 5 4 3 2 1

The authorized representative in the EU for product safety and compliance is Authorised Rep Compliance Ltd., Ground Floor, 71 Lower Baggot Street, Dublin D02 P593, Ireland. www.arccompliance.com

Text: Kierstie Payge Dolezal
Editor: Avalon Radys
Production editor: Peggy Gannon
Designer: Brielle Stein
Illustrations: Arctic Fever

Library of Congress Cataloging-in-Publication Data is available

This book is for informational and educational purposes. This book is not intended to be a substitute for the medical advice of a licensed physician. The reader should consult with their doctor in any matters relating to their health or before starting a new exercise program.

The information in this book is not intended to treat, diagnose, cure, or prevent disease. This book is not sponsored or endorsed by any organization or company. The information in this book is based on experience and research done by the author. Neither the publisher nor the author accept any liability of any kind for any damages caused, directly or indirectly, from the use of the information in this book.

ISBN: 978-1-63217-624-0

Sasquatch Books
1325 Fourth Avenue, Suite 1025
Seattle, WA 98101

SasquatchBooks.com

Introduction

Welcome—and thank you for being here. My name is Kierstie, and since 2017, I've had the incredible privilege of teaching yoga. In 2019, my journey took a significant shift when I started teaching chair yoga to seniors. What started as a new teaching opportunity quickly became a deep passion and one of the most meaningful callings of my life.

Since then I've worked with seniors in nursing homes, specialty care centers, memory care facilities, and more. I've had the honor of guiding people across a wide spectrum of abilities—from active older adults to those living with partial paralysis, dementia, Alzheimer's, and other chronic conditions. Through all of these experiences, one truth has become beautifully clear: *chair yoga has the power to transform lives, and it can start with just five minutes a day.*

The 5-Minute Promise

Through teaching thousands of seniors, I've learned that the biggest barrier isn't ability—it's getting started. That's why I've built this book on a simple promise: in just five minutes a day, you can begin to improve your strength, balance, flexibility, and confidence.

Throughout these pages, you'll find:

- More than forty-five gentle exercises, including poses, breathing techniques, and meditations
- Clear, step-by-step instructions with modifications for every ability level
- Nine complete sequences that can be completed in five minutes
- Tools to create your own 5-minute practices based on what your body needs that day

Five minutes might not sound like much, but I've watched those minutes add up to profound changes. Eyes light up, bodies grow stronger, and spirits lift. Many of my students naturally extend their practice once they begin, but even if you only have five minutes, you're doing something powerful for yourself.

My Journey to You

When the world changed in 2020 and in-person classes came to a halt, I began filming chair yoga videos from my living room and sharing them online. I had no idea what to expect—but those videos started to reach people far beyond my local community. To date they've been watched by millions of seniors around the world, and I am continually amazed and humbled by the messages I receive from those whose lives have been touched by this practice.

For many of my viewers, chair yoga became more than just exercise—it became a reason to look forward to the day, a way to feel empowered in their bodies again, and a reminder that healing and happiness are always possible, at any age.

What You'll Find in This Book

This book is organized to meet you exactly where you are:

- **PART 1** introduces chair yoga basics—why it works, how to get started safely, and how to make it your own.
- **PART 2** presents individual exercises: breathwork, meditations, and poses for every part of your body (from gentle seated movements to optional standing poses for those ready for more of a challenge).
- **PART 3** brings it all together with complete sequences you can follow.

Whether you're brand-new to yoga or a longtime student looking for a gentler approach, whether you're dealing with limited mobility or you simply want a supported practice, this book will guide you step-by-step.

Your Journey Begins Now

I've written this book from the heart, with deep respect for you and your journey. My greatest hope is that it becomes a tool that you can return to repeatedly to help you live a more fulfilling, joyful, and healthy life.

It's never too late to start to create a kind, loving relationship with your body, your breath, and yourself.

So find a sturdy chair, take a deep breath, and let's begin. Your 5-minute practice starts now.

PART 1

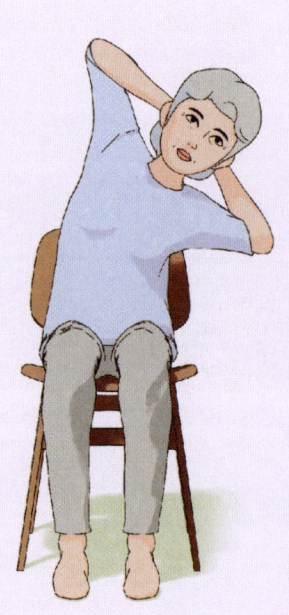

YOUR INTRODUCTION
TO CHAIR YOGA

Why Chair Yoga?

Chair yoga is a gentle and accessible form of movement that brings the benefits of traditional yoga to people of all ages, body types, and mobility levels. Whether you're recovering from injury, spending many hours sitting, or simply looking for a supportive way to move your body, chair yoga can meet you exactly where you are—and it only takes five minutes to start feeling the benefits.

We do chair yoga because it's *effective*, *empowering*, and *inclusive*. It offers a safe and supported way to improve flexibility, build strength, and increase balance without needing to get up and down from the floor. And perhaps even more importantly, it helps us reconnect with our bodies, minds, and breath in a compassionate, nonjudgmental way.

The Benefits Add Up

During my years of teaching, I've discovered that just five minutes of intentional movement can create remarkable changes.

PHYSICAL BENEFITS

- Improved posture and spinal mobility
- Better circulation and joint flexibility
- Increased muscle strength and balance
- Relief from stiffness and everyday aches
- Enhanced coordination and body awareness

COGNITIVE AND EMOTIONAL BENEFITS

- Reduced stress and anxiety
- Improved focus and mental clarity
- Boosted mood and energy levels
- Greater self-confidence
- Better sleep quality

The beauty of chair yoga is that these benefits compound. Five minutes today becomes ten minutes next week. A simple stretch leads to better balance. One deep breath becomes a tool for calm that you carry everywhere.

Your 5-Minute Foundation

Getting started with chair yoga is simple. This is everything you need:

EQUIPMENT

- A sturdy chair without wheels (preferably without armrests)
- Comfortable clothing that allows movement
- Bare feet or grippy socks (shoes are fine too if needed)
- Optional: a small cushion or folded blanket for support

SETTING YOURSELF UP

1. Choose a quiet spot where you won't be interrupted.
2. Sit near the front edge of your chair.
3. Place your feet flat on the floor, hip-width apart.
4. Rest your hands on your thighs.
5. Take three deep breaths—you're ready!

THE PERFECT TIME

While mornings often work well to set a positive tone for the day, the best time is whatever works for *you*. Many of my students love these quick practice times:

- First thing in the morning to wake up your body
- Mid-afternoon to combat the 3 p.m. slump
- Before bed to release the day's tension
- Anytime you need a reset (even at your desk!)

SAFETY FIRST, ALWAYS

Your safety and comfort are paramount. Please remember:

- Listen to your body—if something doesn't feel right, don't do it.
- Move slowly with control and intention.
- Never force any movement or stretch.
- Keep breathing steadily throughout.
- Check with your healthcare provider if you have health conditions or concerns.

Every pose in this book includes modifications because every body is different. What works for one person might need adjustment for another, and that's perfectly normal.

The Power of Your Breath

Breath is at the heart of chair yoga. Your breath is your guide—it helps regulate your nervous system, focus your mind, and connect you to the present moment. Inhale slowly and deeply through your nose, and exhale fully. Try to match your breath with your movement. A steady breath keeps your practice safe, centered, and effective.

Try this now: Inhale slowly through your nose for four counts. Exhale through your nose for four counts. That's it—you've just done your first chair yoga practice!

And remember: You don't have to do it alone. Practicing chair yoga with a friend or in a group can be motivating and fun. Community adds joy to the journey.

Making It Your Own

One of the most important things to remember about chair yoga is that it's *your* practice. We all have different needs, and something that feels right for one person might not work for another. That's not only okay—it's expected.

You should always feel free to adapt poses, sequences, and breathing techniques to meet your unique needs. You might want to modify a pose if you have limited mobility or joint pain or you are recovering from surgery. You can use props such as cushions, yoga blocks, or resistance bands to make movements more accessible or supportive.

For example, if a twist feels too intense, you can reduce your range of motion or simply turn your head. If reaching overhead isn't comfortable, keep your arms lower. There's no one right way to move—only what feels right for you on that particular day.

Some days, you may feel strong and energized; other days, you might need something gentler. Trust that your body knows what it needs, and let your practice reflect that.

If you ever feel unsure, it's a good idea to check in with a healthcare provider, yoga teacher, or physical therapist. They can help tailor your practice and ensure that you're staying safe and supported.

How to Use This Book

This book is designed to be a practical, encouraging guide to help you build your chair yoga practice step-by-step. You'll find meditation, breathing techniques, and individual poses, with clear instructions and modifications. Following the individual exercises are sequences that combine multiple poses into short, themed practices that you can follow.

This book offers three ways to practice:

1. **INDIVIDUAL POSES (PART 2):** Pick one or two exercises that address what you need that day. Tight shoulders? Stiff hips? Low energy? There's a pose to help with all of those.
2. **5-MINUTE SEQUENCES (PART 3):** Follow our ready-made sequences that are designed to fit perfectly into five minutes.
3. **CREATE YOUR OWN:** Mix and match poses to build your own 5-minute practice. Start with a breathing exercise, add three or four poses, and end with a moment of stillness.

REMEMBER: You don't have to do everything. You don't have to be perfect. You just have to begin.

Your Daily 5-Minute Challenge

Here's my challenge to you: *Commit to just five minutes a day for one week.* That's it.

Mark it on your calendar. Set a gentle reminder. Put this book by your favorite chair. Five minutes is less time than it takes to make a cup of tea, yet it can change how your body feels for the entire day.

Most people find that once they start, they naturally want to continue—perhaps for ten or fifteen minutes. But even just five minutes a day can build a habit that supports your body, mind, and spirit.

You now have everything you need to begin your chair yoga journey. In the next section, you'll find a treasury of poses, breathing exercises, and meditations to explore. Take your time. Be patient with yourself. Celebrate small victories.

REMEMBER: Every expert was once a beginner. Every journey starts with a single breath. Your body is wise, and it's been waiting for you to listen. Let's begin.

Definitions

Before we explore the postures and sequences, it's important to first define a few key terms.

Foundational Concepts

- **YOGA:** an ancient practice that unites body, breath, and mind to create balance, awareness, and equanimity. More than physical movement, yoga is a path toward self-discovery, helping quiet the mind, open the heart, and connect with a deeper sense of self and union with all things.

- **EQUANIMITY:** a calm and balanced state of mind, especially during stress or challenge. It's the ability to stay steady, centered, and non-reactive, irrespective of what's happening around you.

- **MINDFULNESS:** paying attention to the present moment with curiosity and kindness, free from judgment.

- **PROPRIOCEPTION:** your body's ability to sense where it is in space, helping with balance, movement, and coordination.

- **AWARENESS:** noticing what's happening inside and around you—your thoughts, feelings, bodily sensations, and environment.

- **MEDITATION:** a practice of focusing the mind to build awareness, calm, and clarity.

- **AFFIRMATIONS:** positive statements that you repeat to shift your mindset and reinforce beliefs.

- **VISUALIZATION:** using your imagination to create mental images for relaxation, focus, or goal-setting.

Breathing Terms

- **UJJAYI (OO-JAI):** a yoga breathing technique in which you slightly constrict your throat to create an ocean-like sound, helping to calm and focus the mind.

Body/Movement Terms

- **DORSIFLEXION:** bending the foot upward toward the shin (such as when you flex your toes upward).

- **ISOMETRIC:** a type of exercise in which muscles contract without moving the joint (such as holding a plank position).

- **SUN SALUTATION:** a flowing sequence of yoga poses used to warm up the body and connect breath to movement.

- **FLEXION:** bending a joint (such as bringing your knee toward your chest).

- **EXTENSION:** straightening a joint (such as stretching your leg out backward).

Systems

- **LYMPHATIC SYSTEM:** part of your immune system that moves fluid through the body, helping to clear waste and fight infection.

- **RESPIRATORY SYSTEM:** the system that helps you breathe, bringing in oxygen and removing carbon dioxide.

- **CARDIOVASCULAR SYSTEM:** your heart and blood vessels, working together to transport blood, oxygen, and nutrients throughout your body.

- **ENERGETIC SYSTEM:** the flow of energy (such as *prana* or *chi*) through the body in yoga and holistic practices, often linked to chakras or meridians.

- **NERVOUS SYSTEM:** the body's communication system, consisting of the brain, spinal cord, and nerves. It controls everything from movement to emotions.

- **PARASYMPATHETIC:** the "rest and digest" system; it calms the body and supports recovery.

- **SYMPATHETIC:** the "fight or flight" system; it activates during stress or danger.

PART 2

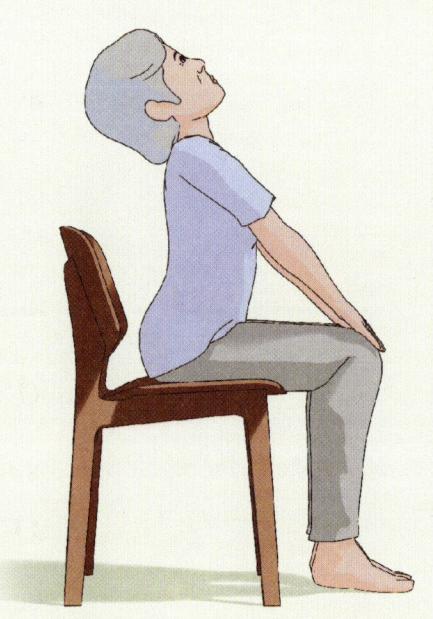

The Exercises: Simple Movements for Every Body

This section contains over forty-five exercises—including meditations, breathing practices, and yoga poses—all designed to help you build strength, find calm, and feel better in just five minutes a day.

How to Use This Section

Think of this as your personal menu of movements. You can:
- Pick and choose individual exercises based on what you need.
- Follow the 5-minute combinations suggested throughout.
- Create your own 5-minute practice by combining three to five exercises

Each exercise includes:
- Clear, step-by-step instructions
- Tips for best results
- Modifications to make it easier or more challenging
- Helpful "Add-Ons" for variety

Your Complete Exercise Collection

Start with Stillness: Meditation and Breathwork

These practices calm your mind and prepare your body.
Perfect for beginning or ending any session.

- **Four meditation practices**
- **Four breathing exercises**

Gentle Movement: Seated Poses

From head to toe, these seated movements improve flexibility, strength, and circulation—all from the safety of your chair.

- **Full body poses** (Poses 1–15)
- **Lower body poses** (Poses 16—22)
- **Upper body and core poses** (Poses 23–30)
- **Head, neck, and shoulders** (Poses 31–36)

Optional Advanced: Standing Poses

Standing poses use your chair for support while building balance and strength.

- **Supported standing balancing** (Poses 37–45)

REMEMBER: You don't need to master every exercise. Start with what feels good, and your practice will naturally grow.

Meditation Practices

Any of these meditations can be your complete 5-minute practice. Or combine them with gentle movement for a balanced session.

MEDITATION 1: Breath Awareness (*Anapana*)

Type: Mindfulness and Awareness
Focus: Calm, clarity, present-moment awareness

Overview: Anapana is a breath awareness practice that centers the mind by focusing on the natural breath. It's a gentle, grounding way to build mindfulness and ease mental chatter. Perfect for calming anxiety, finding focus, or starting your day.

Instructions:

1. Bring your attention to the breath as it flows in and out through your nose.
2. Notice the sensation of air at the nostrils—cool as you inhale, warm as you exhale.
3. If your mind wanders, gently return to your breath.
4. Continue for up to ten minutes.

Tip:
Don't control the breath—just observe it. Let it be natural and effortless.

Modifications:
Start with 1–2 minutes. Use a timer or count breaths if that helps you stay focused.

MEDITATION 2: Visualization

Type: Relaxation and Focus
Focus: Creativity, clarity, emotional healing

Overview: Visualization meditation involves creating a mental image to help calm the mind and body. It's a powerful way to shift focus, reduce stress, and promote positive emotions. Great for stress relief, goal-setting, or a midday reset.

Instructions:

1. Sit comfortably, close your eyes, and relax.
2. Take a few deep breaths to settle your mind.
3. Visualize a peaceful scene (such as a beach or forest) or a specific goal.
4. Engage your senses—see, hear, and feel the scene vividly.
5. If your mind wanders, gently bring it back to your image.
6. Continue for 5–10 minutes.

Tip:
Choose a positive, calming image to deepen relaxation. The more detail, the better.

Modifications:
Start with simple images, such as sunsets or flowing water, and build up to more complex scenes.

MEDITATION 3: Loving Kindness (*Metta*)

Type: Heart-Centered Meditation
Focus: Compassion, emotional balance, connection

Overview: Metta cultivates feelings of love, compassion, and goodwill—first toward yourself, then toward others. It's a beautiful practice for difficult days, relationship stress, or building self-compassion.

Instructions:

1.   Sit comfortably with your eyes closed, and breathe gently.
2.   Start by silently repeating phrases such as *"May I be happy. May I be peaceful. May I be free."*
3.   After a few minutes, extend the phrases to include others.
     For example:
     - People you love
     - Neutral people
     - Difficult people
     - All beings everywhere
4.   Breathe with each phrase, allowing the feelings to grow.

Tip:
If it feels hard at first, that's okay—just stay with the words and let your heart open in its own time

Modifications:
Use your own phrases that feel meaningful. Start with just yourself and one other person.

MEDITATION 4: Affirmation Meditation (*Mantra*)

Type: Mindset and Intention
Focus: Confidence, clarity, self-worth

Overview: Mantra combines breath awareness with positive statements to shift your mindset and anchor into your intentions. It's powerful for boosting confidence, calming the mind, and reprogramming negative thought patterns.

Instructions:

1. On each inhale, silently say a positive affirmation (e.g., *"I am calm"*).
2. On each exhale, let go of any doubt or tension (e.g., *"I release stress"*).
3. Repeat the same affirmation or switch it up based on what you need.
4. Continue for a few minutes, syncing your words with your breath.

Tip:
Choose affirmations that feel true or supportive and are short, simple, and meaningful.

Modifications:
Speak the affirmations silently or out loud. Write your own or choose a theme (such as courage, peace, or self-love).

5-MINUTE MEDITATION MENU

Choose from these calming combinations when you need mental clarity, emotional balance, or a peaceful pause in your day. Each blend is designed to shift your state of mind in just five minutes.

- Morning Clarity: Breath Awareness (3 min) + Affirmation (2 min)
- Stress Buster: Visualization (5 min)
- Heart Opener: Loving Kindness (5 min)
- Quick Reset: any single practice (5 min)

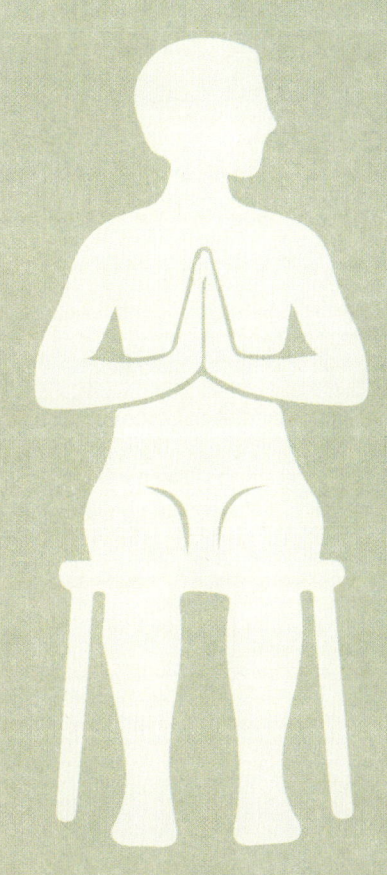

Breathwork Practices

These exercises are perfect for a 5-minute reset and a dose of stress relief anytime you need it. Try combining two to three techniques for a complete respiratory reset.

BREATHWORK 1: Square Breathing

Type: Grounding Technique
Focus: Calm, breath awareness, nervous system balance

Overview: Square Breathing is a simple practice to calm the mind and body by using equal counts for each part of the breath: inhale, hold, exhale, hold. It's great for reducing stress, improving focus, and creating a sense of inner balance. I love to practice Square Breathing whenever I'm feeling anxious and stressed. Even five rounds (about two minutes) can shift your nervous system from stressed to settled.

Instructions:

1. Sit upright in a chair, with your feet flat and your hands resting on your thighs.
2. Inhale through your nose for a count of 4.
3. Hold your breath for 4.
4. Exhale through your nose for 4.
5. Hold the breath out for 4.
6. Repeat for 4–8 rounds.

Tip:
Visualize drawing a square—one side per breath phase—to stay focused.

Modifications:
Start with 3-count breaths if needed. Add a cushion behind your back or under your feet for support.

BREATHWORK 2:
Alternate Nostril Breathing (*Nadi Shodhana*)

Type: Balancing and Centering Technique
Focus: Nervous system regulation, mental clarity, emotional balance

Overview: Nadi Shodhana is a calming breath technique used to harmonize the left and right hemispheres of the brain. It helps reduce stress, clear the mind, and bring your body into a more balanced, grounded state. I love turning to this practice when I need to reset my energy or feel more focused and present.

Instructions:

1. Bring your right hand to your face. Rest your index and middle fingers between your eyebrows.
2. Use your thumb to gently close your right nostril. Inhale through the left nostril slowly and fully.
3. Close the left nostril with your ring finger, then release the thumb and exhale through the right nostril.
4. Inhale through the right nostril.
5. Close the right nostril with your thumb, open the left, and exhale through the left nostril.
6. That's one round. Repeat for 4–8 rounds.

Tip:
Focus on the sensation of air flowing in and out. Let your breath be smooth and even—don't use any force. This is a great practice before meditation or when you're winding down for sleep.

Modifications:
If the finger placement feels awkward, rest your hand lightly on your lap and simply visualize the breath flowing through alternate nostrils.

BREATHWORK 3: Breath Retention

Type: Nervous System Reset
Focus: Calm, control, inner stillness

Overview: Breath Retention is a simple yet powerful technique that builds awareness, control, and resilience. By gently holding the breath after an inhale, you can create a moment of stillness that helps to reset the nervous system, sharpen focus, and promote a deep sense of calm. I love using this practice when I need to feel more grounded and centered—especially before a big task or during a stressful moment. It also helps build resilience and reset energy.

Instructions:

1. Inhale slowly through your nose (4–5 seconds).
2. Hold the breath in for 5 seconds.
3. Exhale slowly through your nose (5–6 seconds).
4. Optional: take a brief pause before the next inhale.
5. Repeat for 4–8 rounds.

Tip:
During the hold, imagine stillness—such as a calm lake.

Modifications:
Start with a 3-second hold if needed. Let it feel gentle, not forced.

BREATHWORK 4: Yogic Breath (*Ujjayi*)

Type: Energizing and Calming
Focus: Breath control, presence, nervous system balance

Overview: Ujjayi (pronounced oo-jai) is a warming, oceanic-sounding breath used to focus the mind and steady the nervous system. It's great for both energizing and calming, depending on how it's used. It is often considered the "yoga breath" and can be used as a tool during your practice to keep you present and focused.

Instructions:

1. Inhale deeply through your nose.
2. Exhale through your nose while gently constricting the back of your throat (like fogging a mirror, but with your mouth closed).
3. Keep the breath smooth and steady.
4. Continue for 4–8 rounds or a few minutes.

Tip:
Listen for the soft "ocean wave" sound to stay focused and present.

Modifications:
Start with just the exhale if the inhale feels tricky. Keep the throat gentle—don't strain.

5-MINUTE BREATHING BREAKS

These breath combinations work like a reset
button for your nervous system. Perfect when
you need quick stress relief, improved focus,
or an energy shift—no movements are required.

- Instant Calm: Square Breathing (5 min)
- Balance Builder: Alternate Nostril Breathing (3 min) +
Breath Retention (2 min)
- Energy Boost: Yogic Breath (2 min) + Breath Retention (3 min)

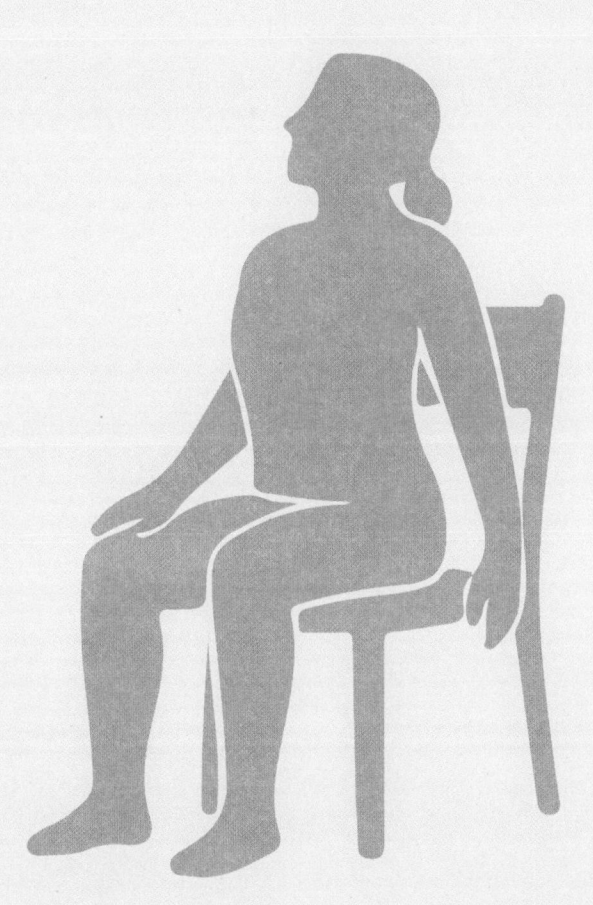

Full Body Poses

POSE 1: Seated Equal Pose (*Samasthiti*)

Type: Grounding Posture
Main Focus: Posture alignment, balance
Secondary Focus: Spine, shoulders, mindfulness

Overview: Samasthiti is a grounding posture that represents a "new beginning" or "fresh start" and promotes physical alignment and balance. It encourages proper posture, cultivating a sense of equanimity in the mind. Practicing this pose helps to center your body and mind, fostering focus and calm, especially before or after a yoga practice. It is the perfect way to begin every practice.

Instructions:

1. Sit tall in a chair with your feet flat on the floor and your knees aligned with your hips.
2. Rest your hands on your thighs, palms facing down, and relax your shoulders.
3. Engage your core, lengthen your spine, and keep your chin parallel to the floor.
4. Breathe deeply, maintaining this posture for several rounds of breath.

Tip:
Focus on a steady breath to maintain balance and calmness in the body and mind.

Modifications:
For a gentler option, place a cushion or block under your feet for added support.

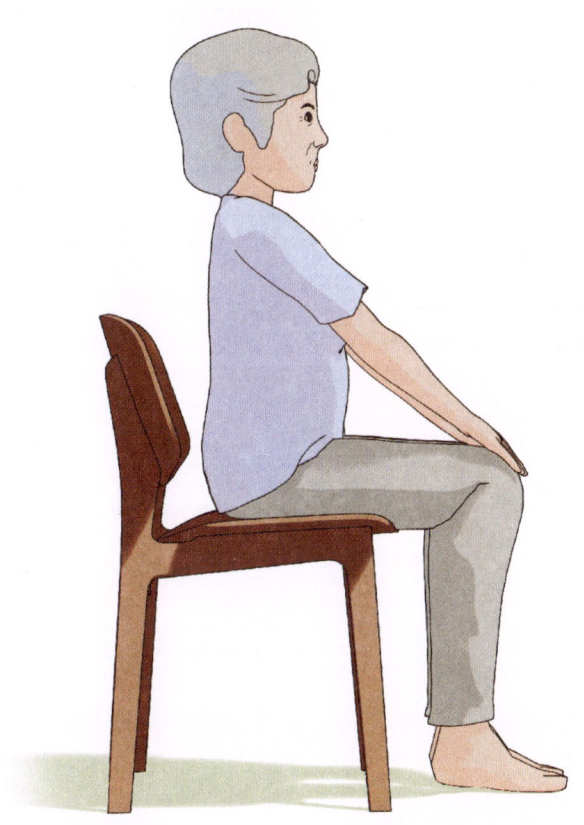

POSE 2: Seated Cow Pose

Type: Spinal Extension
Main Focus: Spine, chest, posture
Secondary Focus: Neck, shoulders

Overview: Seated Cow Pose gently opens the front body and encourages healthy spinal extension. Ideal for counteracting slouched posture, this pose increases circulation and brings energy into the upper body—especially helpful for those who spend a lot of time sitting.

Instructions:

1. Sit tall in your chair with your feet flat on the floor and your knees aligned with your hips.
2. Rest your hands on your thighs or knees.
3. As you inhale, press your hands into your legs, arch your back slightly, lift your chest, and gently gaze upward.
4. Pull your shoulders down and back, creating space across your chest.
5. Hold for a breath, or flow into Seated Cat Pose (page 26) on your exhale.

Tip:
Keep the shoulders soft and let the movement come from your spine—not just your neck.

Modifications:
If your neck feels strained, keep your gaze forward or slightly downward instead of lifting your head.

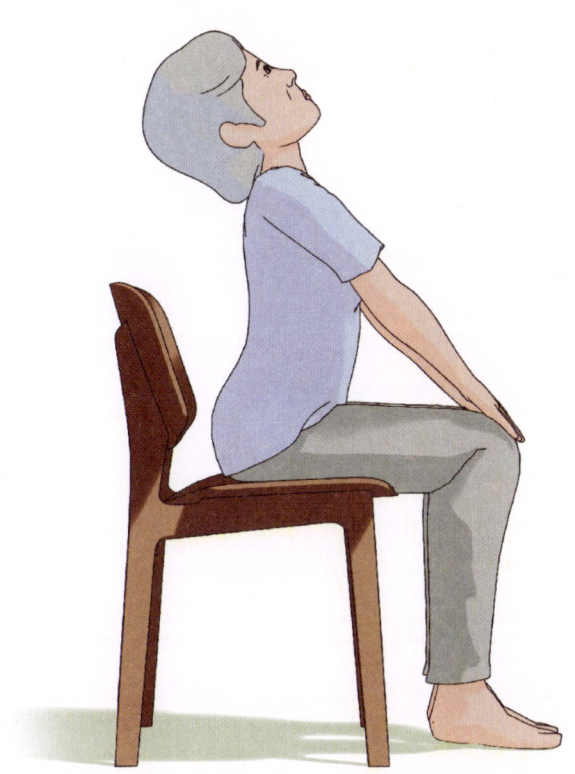

POSE 3: Seated Cat Pose

Type: Spinal Flexion
Main Focus: Spine, core
Secondary Focus: Upper back, neck

Overview: Seated Cat Pose encourages spinal flexion and is a wonderful way to release tension in the back of your body. It promotes flexibility, core engagement, and emotional release, making it a great grounding pose during any seated sequence.

Instructions:

1. Sit tall in your chair with your feet flat on the floor and your knees aligned with your hips.
2. Rest your hands on your thighs or knees.
3. Exhale, then round your spine, draw your belly in, and tuck your chin toward your chest.
4. Feel the stretch across your upper back and between your shoulder blades.
5. Hold for a breath or follow with Seated Cow Pose (page 24) on your next inhale.

Tip:
Engage your abdominal muscles as you round the spine, and keep your movement smooth and intentional.

Modifications:
If needed, reduce the depth of the spinal curve or keep the chin slightly lifted to avoid straining the neck.

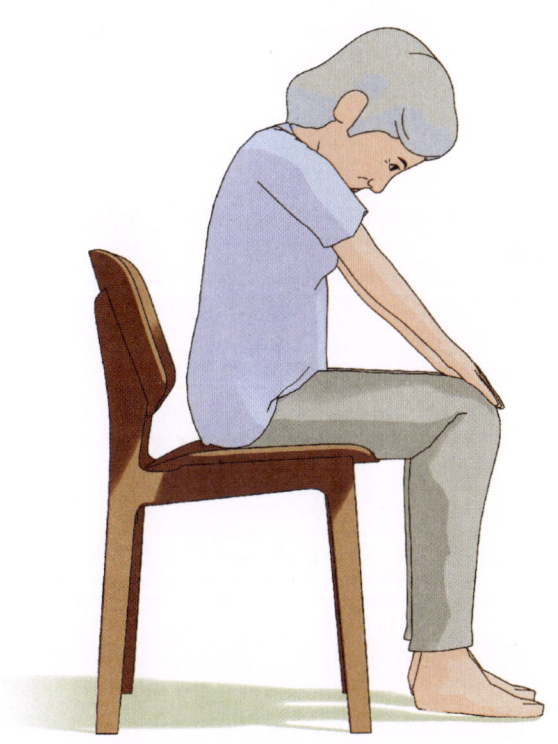

POSE 4: Seated Extended Mountain Pose

Type: Grounding Posture with Upper Body Stretch
Main Focus: Posture, alignment, upper body stretch
Secondary Focus: Shoulders, arms, spine

Overview: Seated Extended Mountain Pose with your arms up offers an uplifting stretch while promoting proper posture and body alignment. It lengthens the spine and opens the chest, enhancing both physical and mental clarity and focus. This posture is a great way to reset your body and mind. It serves as a strong starting point and can easily be built upon to create a full sequence.

Instructions:

1. Sit tall with your feet flat on the floor and knees aligned with your hips.
2. Rest your hands on your thighs, palms down. Relax your shoulders.
3. As you inhale, extend your arms overhead, palms facing each other and fingers reaching up.
4. Engage your core, lengthen your spine, and hold for several breaths.

Tip:
Keep your arms active by reaching through your fingertips, while keeping your shoulders relaxed and away from your ears.

Modifications:
If you experience shoulder discomfort, keep your arms lower or bend your elbows.

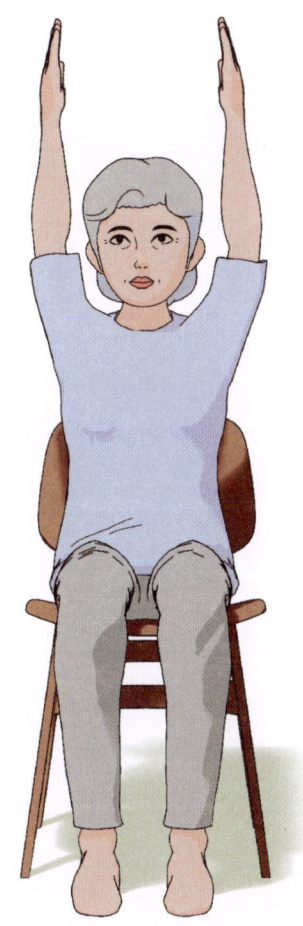

POSE 5: Seated Extended Mountain Pose with a Side Body Stretch

Type: Spinal Mobility and Side Body Extension
Main Focus: Lateral, oblique stretch
Secondary Focus: Legs, shoulders, arms, spine, neck

Overview: Seated Extended Mountain Pose with a Side Body Stretch offers a lateral upper body stretch while promoting mobility and longevity of the spine.

Instructions:

1. Inhale and stretch your arms high.
2. As you exhale, release your right arm down by your side and lean toward your right, stretching your left arm overhead.
3. Extend the stretch down through your fingertips while pushing your left hip further left.
4. Hold for several breaths, feeling the stretch along your side body.
5. Repeat on the opposite side.

Tip:
Engage your core to support your lower back and keep your chest open as you lean to one side. This will help maintain length in your spine and will ensure a deeper, more stable side body stretch.

Modifications:
If you experience shoulder discomfort, keep your arms lower or bend your elbows.

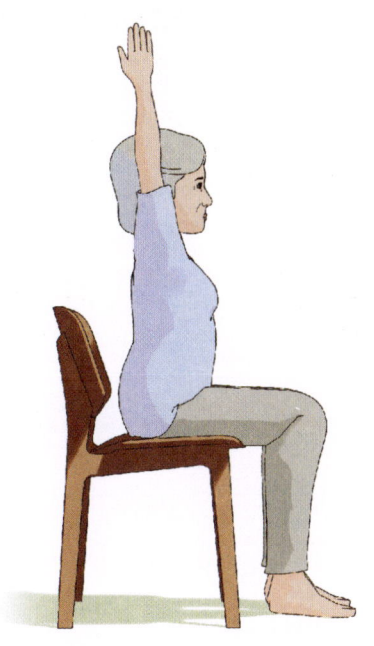

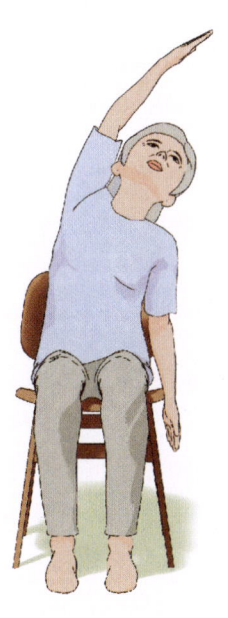 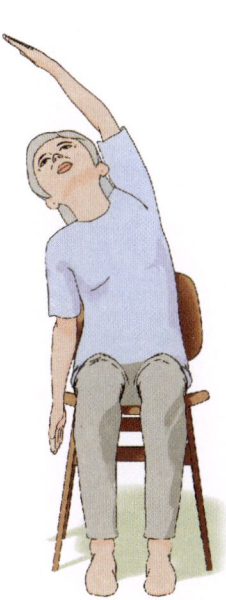

POSE 6: Seated Extended Mountain Pose with a Backbend

Type: Spinal Mobility and Upper Body Extension
Main Focus: Spine, chest, shoulder stretch
Secondary Focus: Legs, arms, neck

Overview: Seated Extended Mountain Pose with a Backbend opens the chest and promotes spinal mobility. It stretches the front body, encourages deeper breathing, and helps improve posture and flexibility.

Instructions:

1. Inhale, stretching your arms high for Seated Extended Mountain Pose.
2. As you exhale, gently arch your back and lift your chest toward the ceiling.
3. Keep your arms active, with the option to bend your elbows out to the sides (like a cactus), reaching upward while gently pressing your hips down.
4. Hold for several breaths, feeling a stretch across your chest and spine.
5. Return to neutral and repeat if desired.

Tip:
Engage your core and avoid over-arching your lower back to protect your spine while deepening the backbend.

Modifications:
To reduce intensity, keep your arms lower or bend your elbows slightly. If you have lower back discomfort, reduce the backbend and focus on lifting through the chest instead.

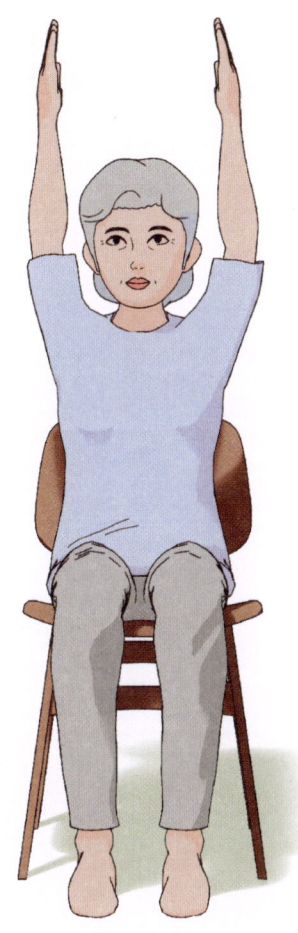
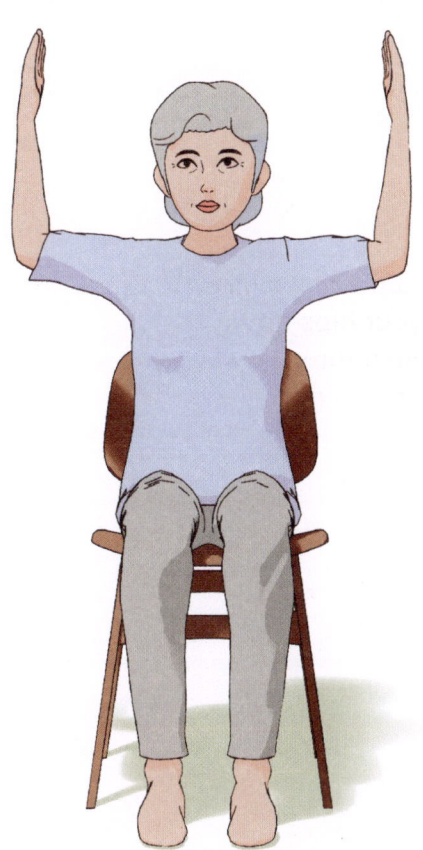

POSE 7: Seated Forward Fold

Type: Hamstring Stretch and Spinal Flexion
Main Focus: Hamstrings, lower back
Secondary Focus: Spine, hips, neck

Overview: Seated Forward Fold stretches your hamstrings and lower back while promoting spinal flexibility and relaxation. This deep fold encourages lengthening in the back of the body and can help relieve tension and improve flexibility over time. It also offers a relaxing bowing sensation that can soothe your nervous system.

Instructions:

1. Sit tall with your feet flat on the floor and your knees aligned with your hips.
2. As you inhale, lengthen your spine.
3. As you exhale, hinge at your hips and fold forward, reaching your hands toward your feet or the floor.
4. Let your head and neck relax, and hold for several breaths.

Tip:
Keep your spine long as you fold, and avoid rounding your back so you deepen the stretch without compromising your posture.

Modifications:
If your hamstrings are tight, move slowly and round your spine more.

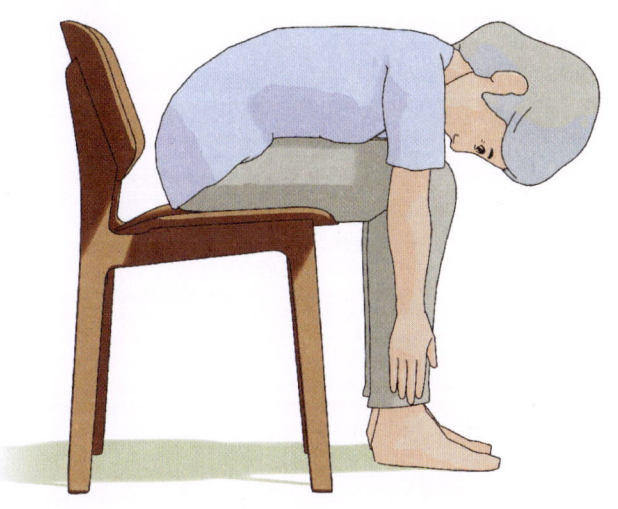

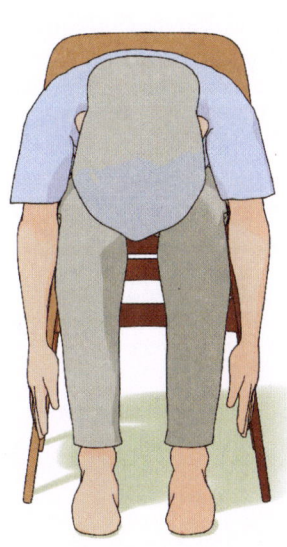

POSE 8: Seated Chair Pose with Hands at Your Heart

Type: Strengthening and Postural Alignment
Main Focus: Legs, core, glutes
Secondary Focus: Spine, shoulders, chest

Overview: This pose strengthens your legs, core, and glutes while promoting focus. Bringing your hands to your heart center encourages an inner connection with self, encouraging self-love and acceptance.

Instructions:

1. Sit tall with your feet flat on the floor and your knees aligned with your hips.
2. Inhale, extend your arms overhead, and bring your palms together. Lower them to meet your heart center.
3. As you exhale, press your feet into the floor and engage your core as you lengthen your spine.
4. For several breaths, keep your spine long, your shoulders relaxed, and your knees over your ankles.

Tip:
Press your palms together at your heart to encourage steadiness and mindfulness while maintaining strength in your legs and core.

Modifications:
To reduce intensity, lower your hands to shoulder height or extend them in front of you.

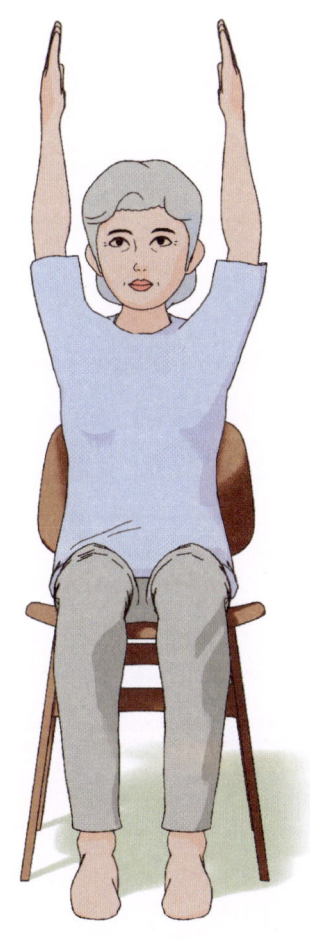
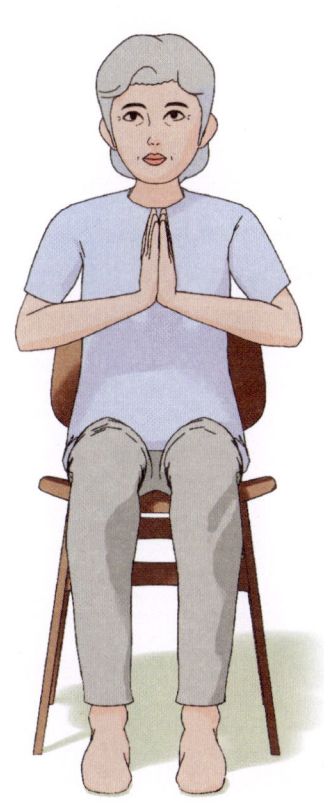

POSE 9: Seated Chair Pose with Open Arm Twists

Type: Spinal Mobility, Upper Body Stretch, and Leg Strengthener
Main Focus: Spinal rotation, shoulders
Secondary Focus: Core, arms, legs, neck

Overview: This pose enhances spinal mobility and leg strength, and is an upper body stretch. This twist improves flexibility, aids in digestion, and promotes better posture by engaging the spine and shoulders.

Instructions:

1. Sit tall with your feet flat on the floor and your knees aligned with your hips.
2. Inhale, extending your arms overhead.
3. As you exhale, twist your torso to one side, lowering one hand to the back of your chair while the other arm extends forward.
4. Keep your spine long and your chest open as you twist, engaging your core for support.
5. Hold for several breaths, then slowly return to the center and repeat on the other side.

Tip:
Engage your core to protect your lower back during the twist, and maintain an open chest throughout.

Modifications:
If twisting is uncomfortable, reduce the range of motion or keep your arms in front of you.

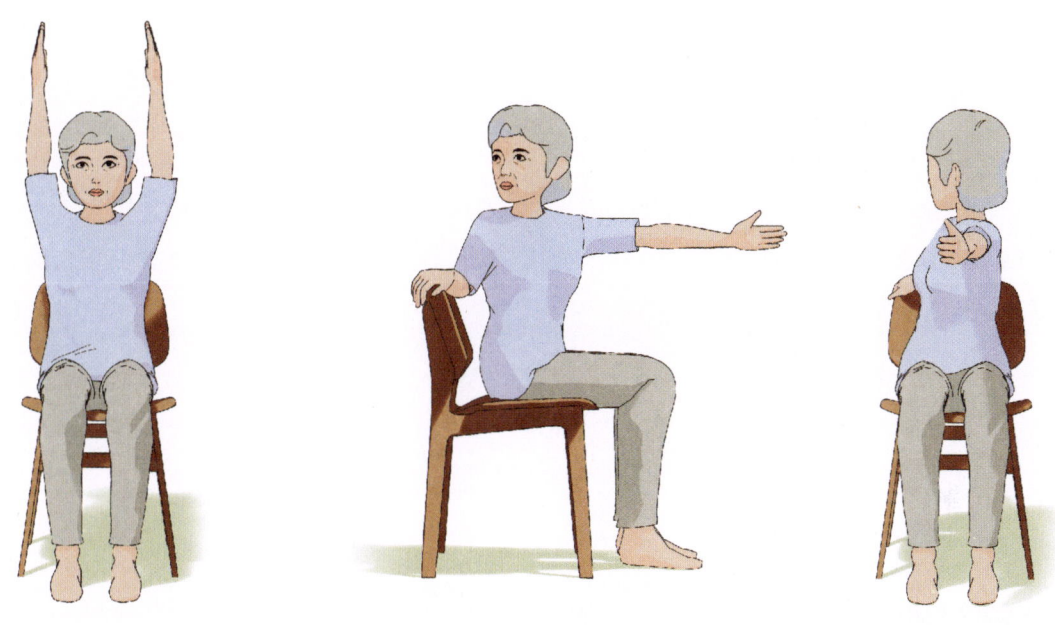

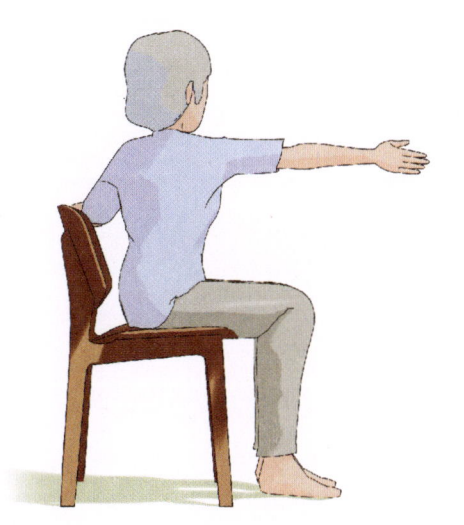

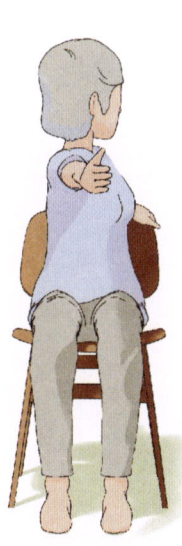

POSE 10: Seated Chair Pose with Oblique Stretch

Type: Lateral Strength and Spinal Flexion
Main Focus: Obliques, side body
Secondary Focus: Core, shoulders, hips, spine

Overview: Seated Chair Pose with Oblique Stretch targets the side of your body, helping to increase strength and mobility in the obliques and spine. This pose stretches the torso and enhances core strength, promoting balance. It can also help with proprioception by moving your body in a unique way.

Instructions:

1. Inhale, extending your arms overhead.
2. As you exhale, bring your hands behind your head and open your elbows wide.
3. Lean to one side, reaching your bottom arm toward your hip and keeping your chest open.
4. Engage your core.
5. Hold for several breaths, then return to the center and repeat on the other side.

Tip:
Keep your hips grounded and engage your core to maintain stability as you stretch to the side.

Modifications:
To reduce intensity, keep your arms lower or bend your elbow during the stretch.

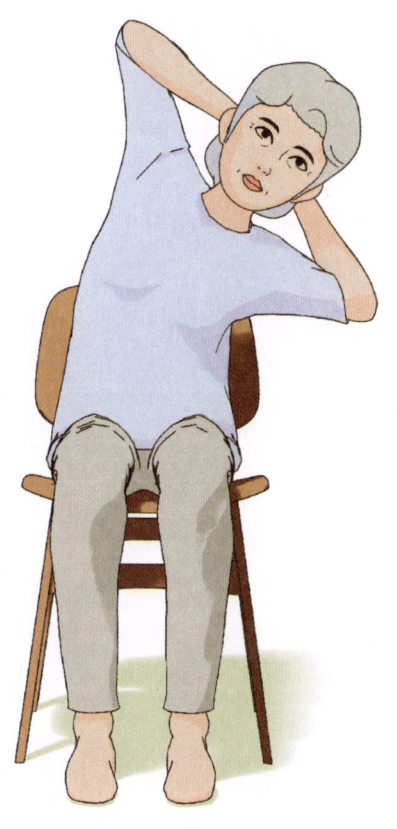
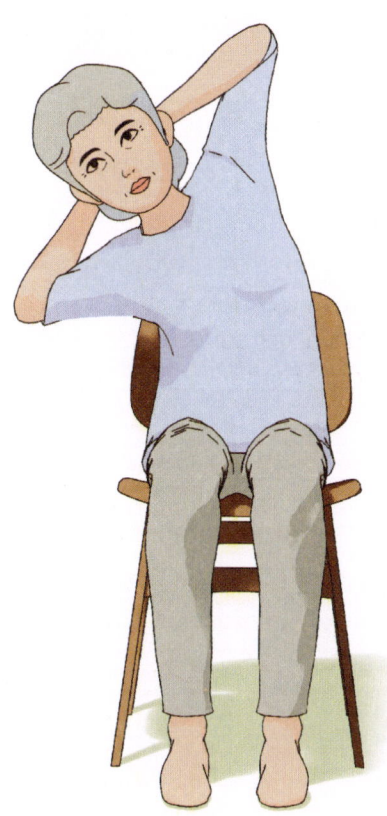

POSE 11: Seated Spinal Twist

Type: Spinal Mobility and Twist
Main Focus: Spine, obliques
Secondary Focus: Shoulders, core, neck

Overview: Seated Spinal Twists help improve spinal mobility, release tension in the back, and stretch the obliques. This pose promotes flexibility in the spine, increases core engagement, and enhances posture.

Instructions:

1. Inhale, extending your arms overhead.
2. As you exhale, twist your torso to one side, bringing one hand to the back of your chair and the other hand to your thigh.
3. Keep your spine long and your shoulders relaxed as you hold the twist, engaging your core.
4. Hold for several breaths, then exhale, return to the center, and repeat on the opposite side.

Tip:
Engage your core and avoid forcing the twist, keeping your chest open and shoulders relaxed.

Modifications:
To reduce intensity, twist to a lesser degree or keep your hands on your thighs without reaching toward the back of the chair.

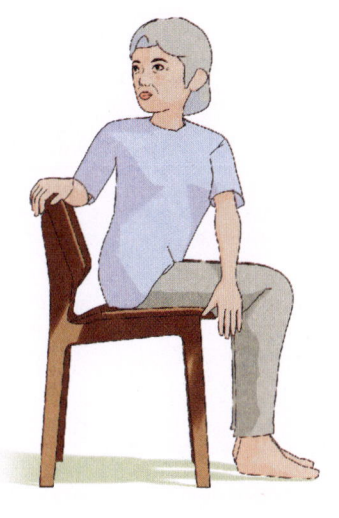

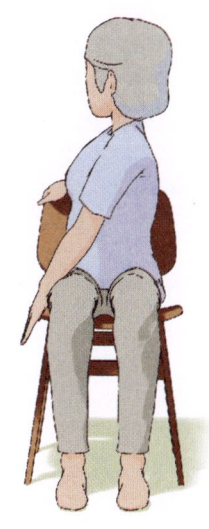

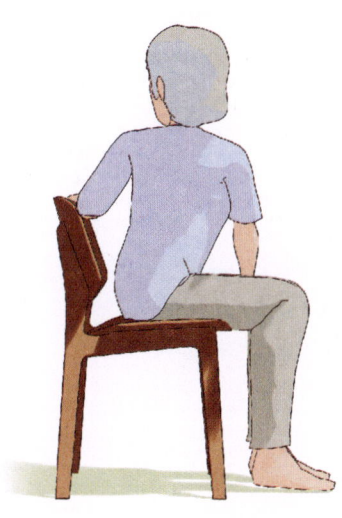

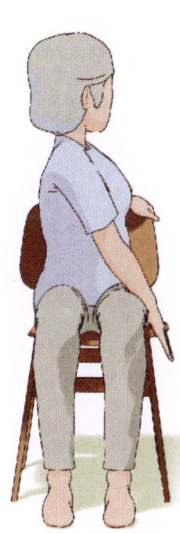

POSE 12: Seated Warrior One (*Virabhadrasana A*)

Type: Hip Opening and Spinal Extension
Main Focus: Hips, legs, chest, spine
Secondary Focus: Shoulders, arms

Overview: Virabhadrasana A strengthens your legs, opens your hips, and encourages spinal extension. This pose promotes stability and balance and stretches the chest, improving posture and overall flexibility.

Instructions:

1. Inhale, extending your arms overhead and bringing your palms together.
2. As you exhale, step one foot to the side and bend your knee, with your foot turned out. Extend your other leg straight in the opposite direction and plant your foot on the floor.
3. Keep your torso upright, engage your core, and gently press your hips forward. Keep your arms lifted.
4. Hold for several breaths, then return to the center and repeat on the other side.

Tip:
Keep your chest open and your hips square to the front to maintain balance and stability in the pose.

Modifications:
To reduce intensity, keep the foot of the straight leg flat on the floor or reduce the range of the lunge. If knee discomfort occurs, adjust the bend of the bent knee.

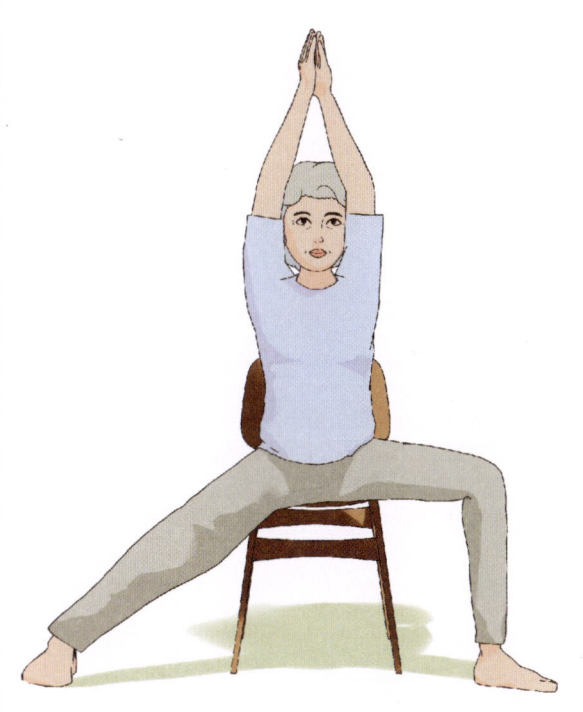

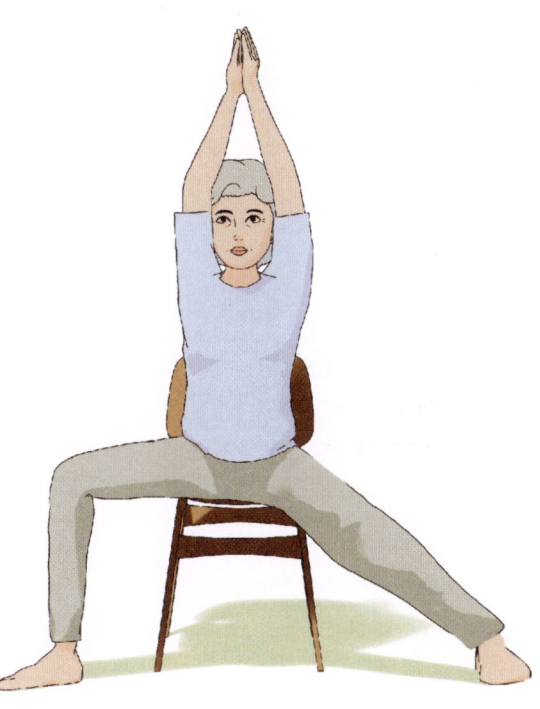

POSE 13: Seated Warrior Two (*Virabhadrasana B*)

Type: Hip Opening and Spinal Extension
Main Focus: Hips, legs, arms, shoulders
Secondary Focus: Spine, chest, neck

Overview: Virabhadrasana B strengthens the legs and arms and opens the chest. It also resembles a fierce and strong Warrior Spirit that encourages a steadfast focus and courage.

Instructions:

1. Inhale, extending your arms out in a T parallel to the floor, palms facing down.
2. As you exhale, step one foot to the side and bend your knee, with your foot turned out. Extend your other leg straight in the opposite direction and plant your foot on the floor.
3. Gaze over your fingertips directly above your bent knee. Keep your torso upright and engage your core.
4. Hold for several breaths and repeat on the other side.

Tip:
Keep your shoulders relaxed, arms extended, and engage your core to maintain stability throughout the pose.

Modifications:
To reduce intensity, decrease the depth of the lunge or keep your arms lower.

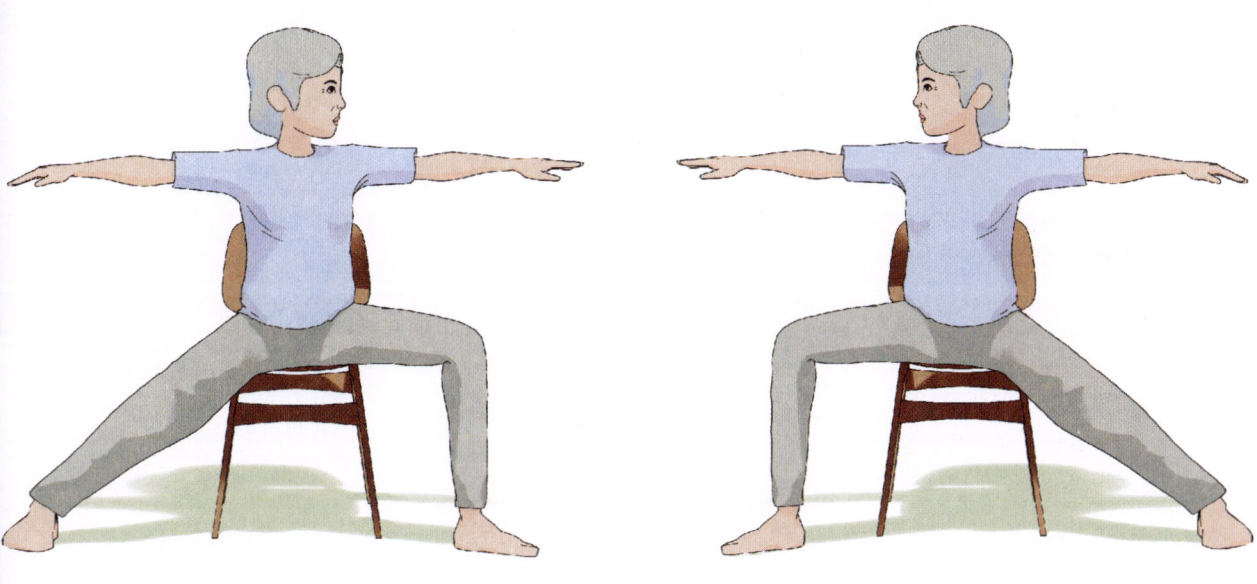

POSE 14: Seated Extended Side Angle

Type: Lateral Stretch and Spinal Extension
Main Focus: Hips, legs, side body
Secondary Focus: Arms, shoulders, spine

Overview: Seated Extended Side Angle stretches the side body, hips, and legs while promoting spinal mobility and flexibility.

Instructions:

1. Begin in a Seated Warrior Two position.
2. Inhale, then exhale. Lower your front elbow to your thigh and extend your back arm toward the ceiling, creating a straight line from hand to heel.
3. Hold for several breaths, feeling the stretch along your side body.
4. Return to the center and repeat on the other side.

Tip:
Engage your core to protect your lower back and maintain balance while deepening the stretch through your side body.

Modifications:
If shoulder discomfort occurs, keep your arm lower or place your hand on your hip. For more support, sit on a cushion or block to elevate your hips.

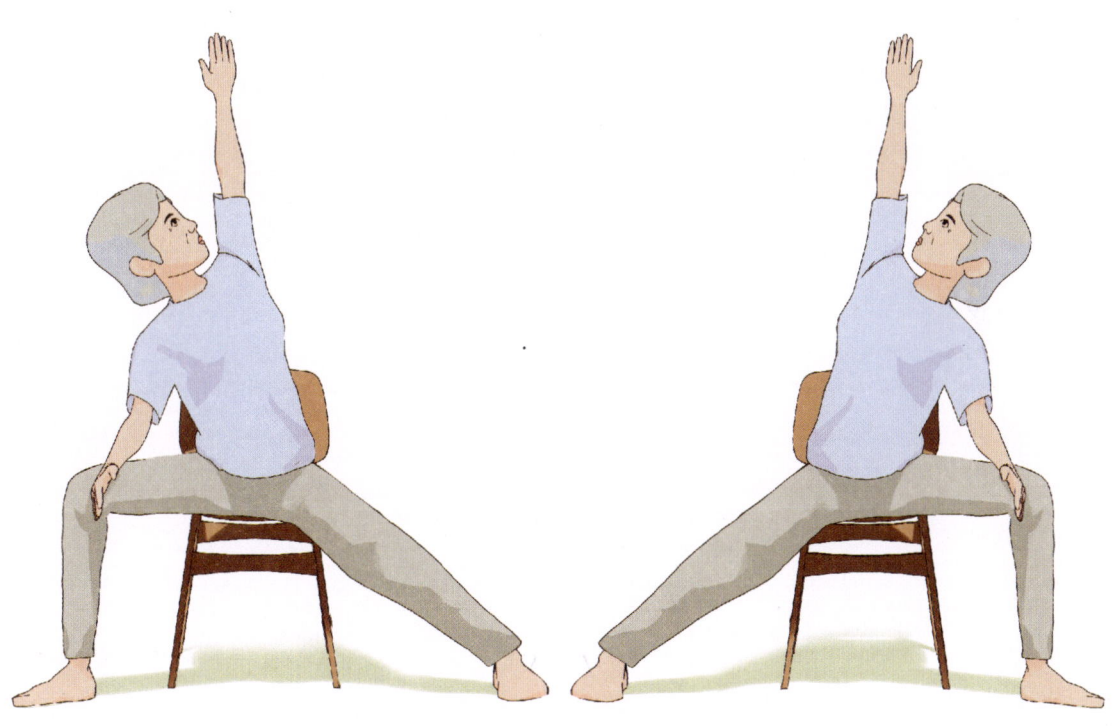

POSE 15: Seated Reverse Warrior

Type: Spinal Extension and Lateral Stretch
Main Focus: Hips, legs, spine
Secondary Focus: Shoulders, arms, side body

Overview: Seated Reverse Warrior stretches the side body while strengthening the legs and promoting spinal flexibility. This pose helps improve posture, stability, and mobility in the hips and spine.

Instructions:

1. Start in a Seated Warrior Two position.
2. As you inhale, release your back hand down to your back leg or the chair and reach your front arm overhead, palm facing up, creating a long line from hand to foot.
3. Hold for several breaths, feeling the stretch along your side body.
4. Return to the center and repeat on the other side.

Tip:
Keep your chest open and shoulders relaxed, while engaging your core to maintain stability and avoid collapsing into your lower back.

Modifications:
To reduce intensity, keep your back hand on your thigh or chair instead of reaching down.

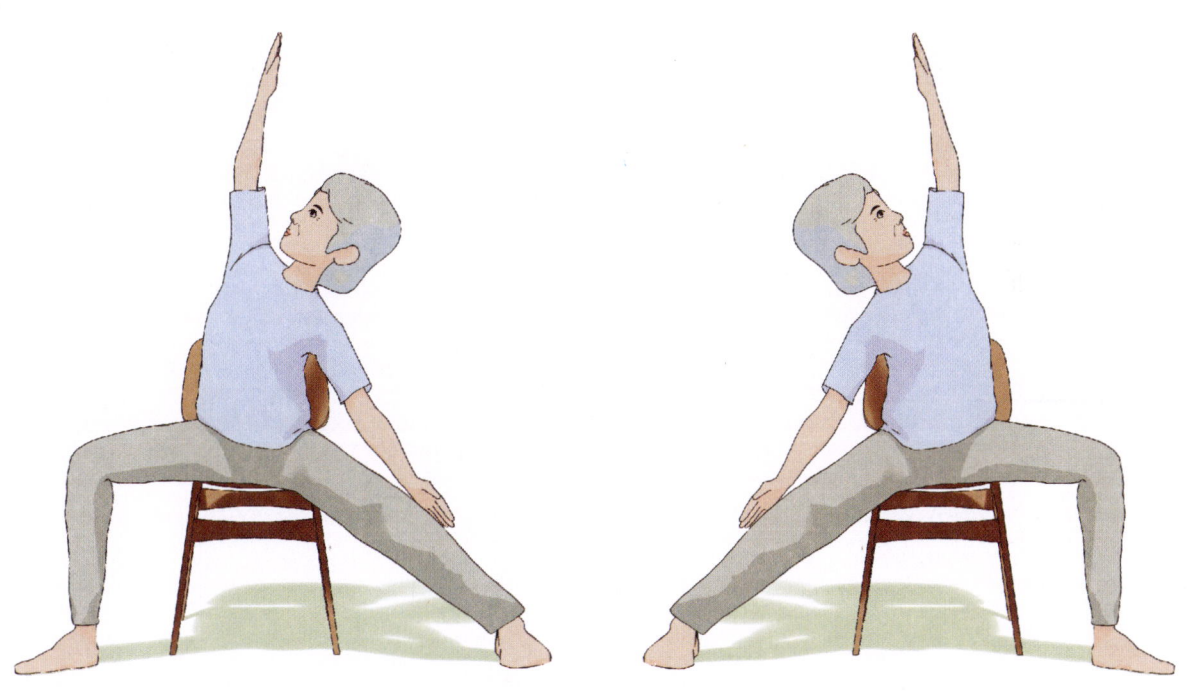

5-MINUTE FULL BODY FLOWS

Wake up your whole body with these balanced sequences that stretch, strengthen, and energize from head to toe. Each flow is a complete mini-practice that leaves you feeling refreshed and ready.

- Morning Energizer
  - Seated Extended Mountain Pose (1 min)
  - Seated Cat-Cow Flow (2 min)
  - Seated Spinal Twist (2 min)

- Warrior Flow
  - Seated Warrior One (1 min each side)
  - Seated Warrior Two (1 min each side)
  - Seated Forward Fold (1 min)

- Gentle Wake-Up
  - Seated Equal Pose (1 min)
  - Seated Extended Mountain Pose with Side Body Stretch (2 min)
  - Seated Chair Pose with Hands at Your Heart (2 min)

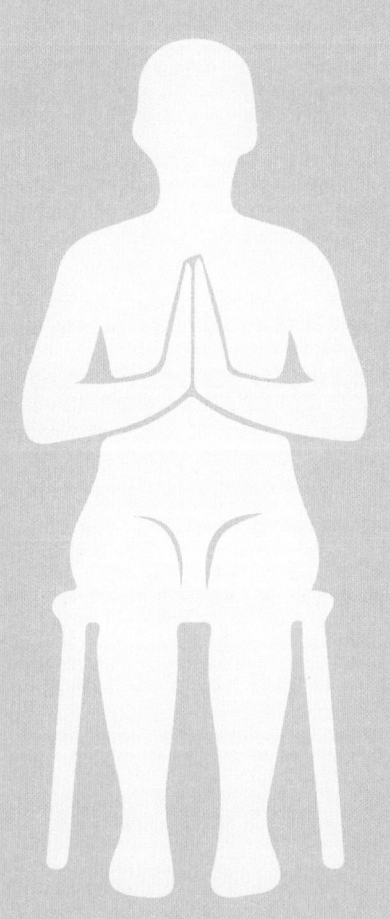

LOWER BODY POSES

POSE 16: Seated Heel Raises and Toe Raises

Type: Strengthening and Mobility
Main Focus: Feet, ankles, calves
Secondary Focus: Legs, core

Overview: Seated Heel Raises and Toe Raises improve ankle mobility, strengthen the calves, and promote balance. This simple exercise helps to enhance circulation and flexibility in the lower legs, which is beneficial for overall foot health.

Instructions:

1. Sit tall with your feet flat on the floor and your knees aligned with your hips.
2. Inhale and raise your heels off the floor, pressing through the balls of your feet.
3. As you exhale, lower your heels back to the floor.
4. Inhale again, lifting your toes off the floor and pressing through your heels.
5. Exhale and lower your toes back down.
6. Repeat the sequence several times, alternating between heel and toe raises.

Tip:
Engage your core to maintain posture and balance while lifting and lowering your heels and toes.

Modifications:
To reduce intensity, perform one movement at a time (either heel or toe raises).

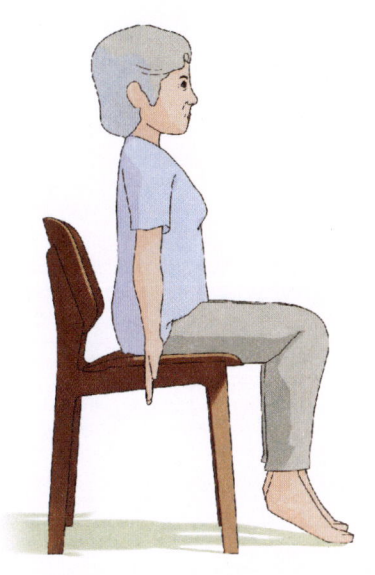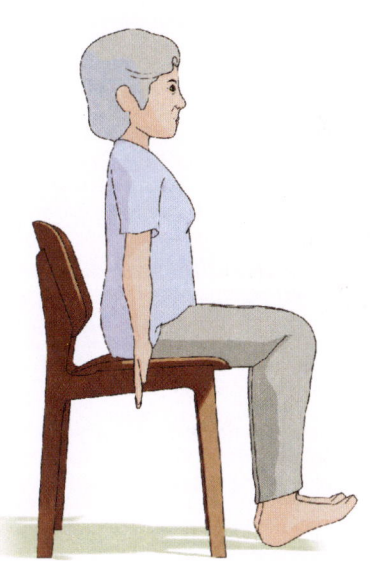

POSE 17: Seated Leg Extension

Type: Strengthening and Mobility
Main Focus: Quadriceps and knees
Secondary Focus: Hips, core

Overview: Seated Leg Extensions strengthen the quadriceps and improve knee joint mobility. This pose helps to enhance leg strength and stability, promoting better posture and balance.

Instructions:

1. Sit tall with your feet flat on the floor and your knees aligned with your hips.
2. As you inhale, extend one leg straight out, keeping your foot flexed and your knee straight.
3. Hold for a few seconds, then exhale and lower your leg back to the floor.
4. Repeat the extension on each side for several rounds.

Tip:
Keep your core engaged to help support your lower back while extending each leg. Focus on keeping your knee straight without locking it.

Modifications:
If extending your leg fully is difficult, only raise it as high as is comfortable.

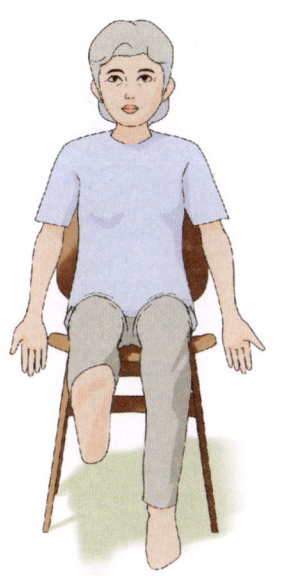
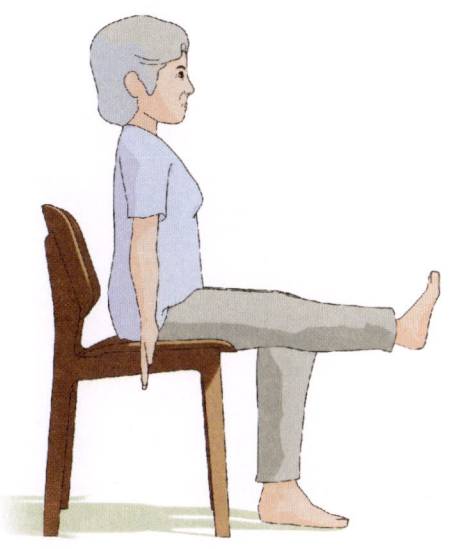

Add-On 1: Seated Leg Extension with Ankle Roll
Keep your leg extended and roll your ankle in a circular motion from left to right to increase ankle mobility. Continue for several rounds, then switch directions. Repeat with the other leg.

Add-On 2: Seated Leg Extension with Flex and Point
Keep your leg extended. Point your toes forward, then dorsiflex your toes back toward you. Repeat several times to strengthen and stretch your ankles. Repeat with the other leg.

Add-On 3: Seated Leg Extension with Isometric Hold
Keep your leg extended and hold for 5–10 breaths to build strength and challenge your abilities. Focus on maintaining a straight leg and engaging your quadriceps throughout. Repeat with the other leg.

POSE 18: Seated Half Wind Removing Pose (Knee to Belly Pose)

Type: Core Activation and Hip Flexion
Main Focus: Core, hips
Secondary Focus: Spine, legs, lower back

Overview: Seated Half Wind Removing Pose gently compresses the abdomen and helps activate the core while offering a mild stretch for the hips. This pose aids in digestion, relieves lower back tension, and strengthens the abdominal muscles.

Instructions:

1. Sit tall with your feet flat on the floor and your knees aligned with your hips.
2. Inhale, lengthening your spine and engaging your core.
3. As you exhale, bring one knee toward your chest and clasp your hands around your shin or knee.
4. Hold for several breaths, then gently release and repeat on the other side.

Tip:
Engage your core as you pull your knee toward your chest to deepen the stretch and protect your lower back.

Modifications:
For a gentler option, keep your foot on the floor and draw the knee in slightly.

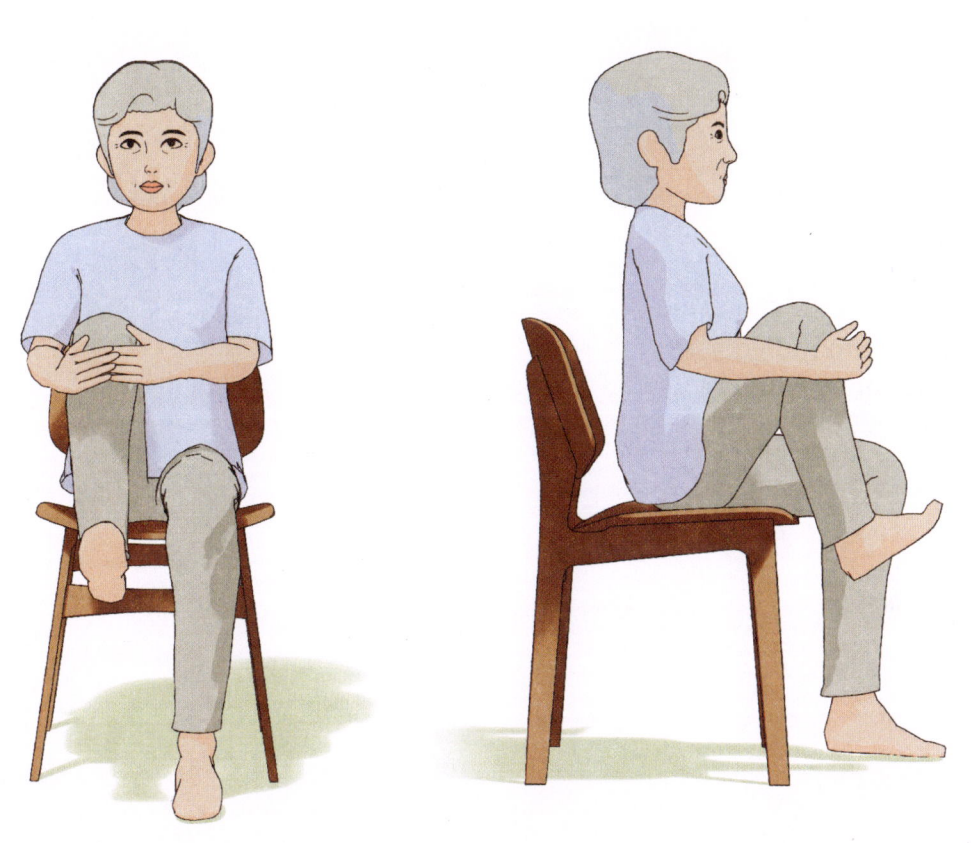

POSE 19: Seated Figure Four

Type: Hip Opener
Main Focus: Hips, external rotation
Secondary Focus: Lower back, IT band (outer thigh), knee mobility

Overview: Hips store tension, particularly in those with sedentary lifestyles, leading to tightness in the IT band, knees, and lower back. Healthy hips are vital for long-term mobility and energy. This figure four stretch improves hip mobility and can be practiced anytime, especially before or after exercise, to enhance movement and reduce discomfort.

Instructions:

1. Interlace your hands around your right knee.
2. Keep your right foot on the ground, lift your left foot, and pull your knee toward your torso.
3. Use your right hand to cross your left ankle over your right knee.
4. Sit tall, gently press the lifted knee for more sensation, and take 5 breaths, then repeat on the other side.

Tip:
Keep your toes in dorsiflexion to protect your knee.

Modifications:
To deepen the figure four stretch, lean forward gradually, reaching for your knee, shin, toes, or floor. For a gentler option, cross your top leg over the bottom as if you were sitting with your legs crossed.

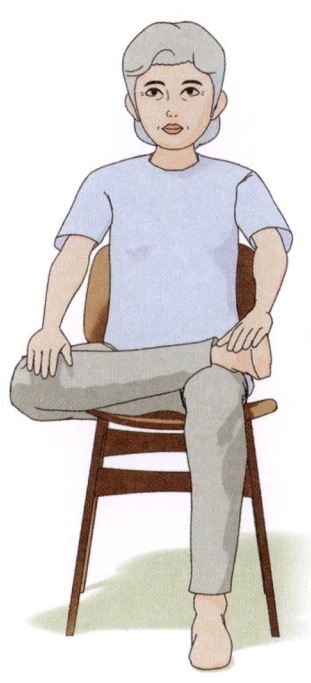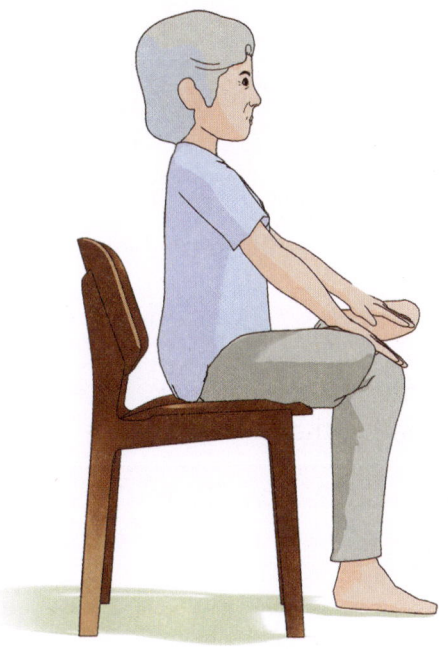

Add-On 1: Seated Figure Four with Twist
While seated in your Figure Four, inhale and raise your arms to the sky. Exhale and twist your torso toward your bent knee, bringing one arm to the outside of your bent knee and the other to the back of your chair.

Add-On 2: Seated Figure Four with Forward Fold
While seated in your Figure Four, inhale and lift your arms high. Exhale and slowly begin to reach your fingertips toward the ground, feeling the stretch in your hips, lower back, and hamstrings.

POSE 20: Seated Shoelace Pose

Type: Hip Opener and Spinal Flexion
Main Focus: Hips, glutes
Secondary Focus: Spine, thighs, lower back

Overview: Seated Shoelace Pose provides a deep stretch to the hips and glutes, while promoting spinal flexibility and releasing tension in the lower back. This pose helps to open the hips and improve mobility, which is beneficial for anyone looking to alleviate stiffness in the lower body.

Instructions:

1. Cross your right leg over your left, with your knees on top of each other.
2. Inhale and lengthen your spine.
3. As you exhale, gently fold forward over your crossed legs.
4. Keep your chest open and your shoulders relaxed as you hold the stretch for several breaths.
5. Return to the center, then repeat on the other side.

Tip:
Engage your core and keep your spine long as you fold forward to deepen the stretch while maintaining a comfortable position.

Modifications:
For a gentler stretch, avoid folding deeply and stay upright with a slight bend in your torso.

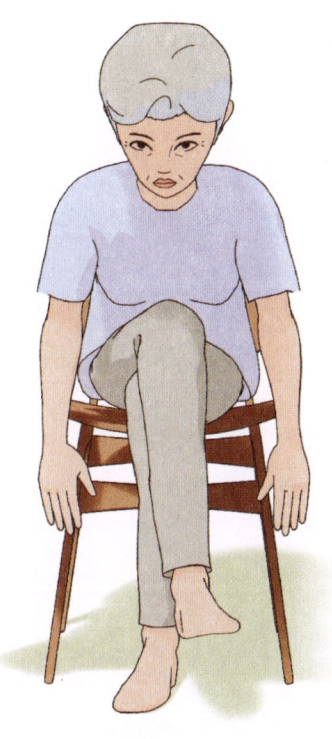

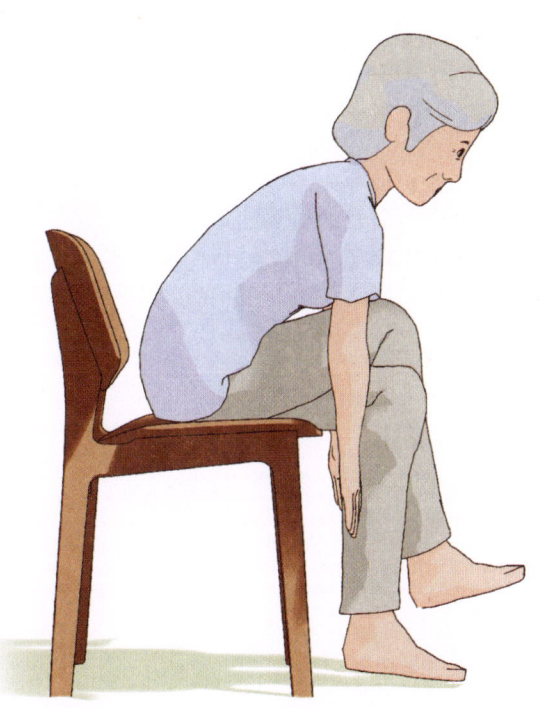

POSE 21: Seated Staff Pose with Both Legs and Arms Lifted

Type: Core Strength and Postural Alignment
Main Focus: Core, legs, shoulders
Secondary Focus: Spine, arms, posture

Overview: Seated Staff Pose with Both Legs and Arms Lifted builds core strength and improves posture by engaging the abdominal muscles and lengthening the spine. This pose helps to enhance overall balance and stability, benefiting both the upper and lower body, and challenges your mind by encouraging you to focus on your breath.

Instructions:

1. Sit tall with your legs extended straight out in front of you, your feet flexed, and your hands resting on the chair by your sides.
2. As you inhale, lengthen your spine and engage your core.
3. Exhale and lift both legs off the floor, keeping them straight and together.
4. Simultaneously, lift both arms overhead, palms facing each other, reaching toward the sky.
5. Hold the pose for several breaths, then gently lower your arms and return to the starting position.

Tip:
Focus on maintaining a long spine, and avoid rounding your back. Engage your core and keep your legs active to maintain balance.

Modifications:
If lifting both legs is challenging, start by lifting one leg at a time or keep your legs on the floor for support. For additional stability, slightly bend your knees as you lift.

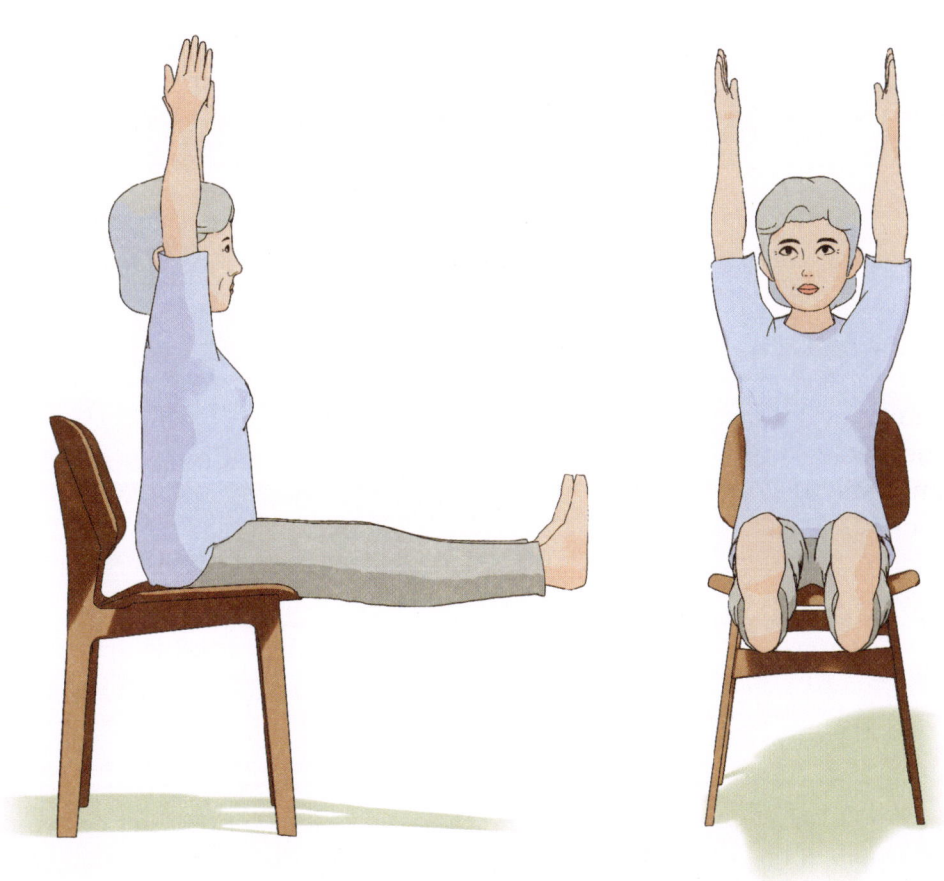

POSE 22: Seated Wide Straddle

Type: Hip Opener and Spinal Lengthening
Main Focus: Hips, inner thighs
Secondary Focus: Spine, core, hamstrings

Overview: Seated Wide Straddle helps to open the hips and stretch the inner thighs while promoting flexibility in the spine. This pose improves posture, increases hip mobility, and gently stretches the legs, offering relief from tightness in the lower body.

Instructions:

1. Sit tall with your legs extended straight in front of you, then widen your legs to a comfortable distance, with your knees bent.
2. Inhale and lengthen your spine.
3. As you exhale, begin to fold forward from your hips.
4. Reach your hands toward the floor or your feet.
5. Hold for several breaths, feeling the stretch in your inner thighs and hamstrings.

Tip:
Keep your feet flexed and active, engaging your inner thighs and core as you fold forward to deepen the stretch while maintaining length through your spine.

Modifications:
For a gentler stretch, bend your knees slightly or stay upright without folding forward.

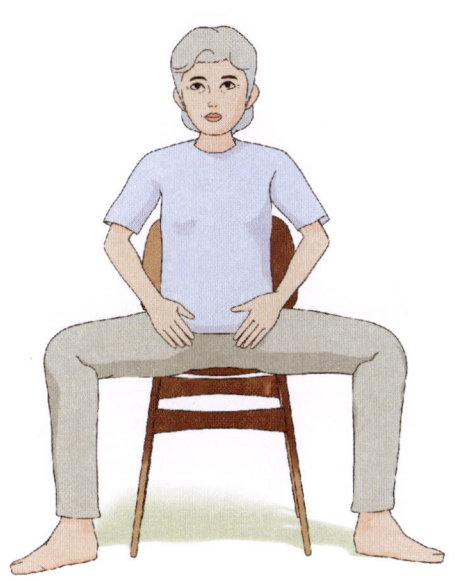
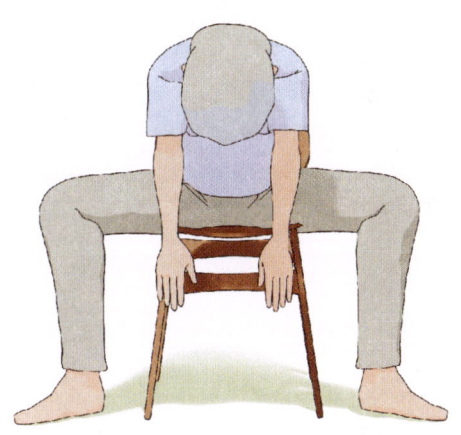

Add-On 1: Seated Wide Straddle with Side Body Stretch
Inhale and lift your arms high toward the sky. Exhale and lower one arm down toward the inside of one leg, extending your fingertips toward your knee. Reach your opposite arm overhead. Inhale, return to the center, and then repeat on the other side.

5-MINUTE LOWER BODY RELIEF

Give your hips, legs, and feet the attention they deserve with these targeted combinations. Perfect for releasing the tension that builds from sitting, walking, or simply living.

- Hip Helper
  - Seated Figure Four (2 min each side)
  - Seated Shoelace Pose (1 min)

- Leg Strengthener
  - Seated Heel Raises and Toe Raises (2 min)
  - Seated Leg Extension with Isometric Hold (3 min)

- Flexibility Flow
  - Seated Half Wind Removing Pose (1 min each side)
  - Seated Wide Straddle (3 min)

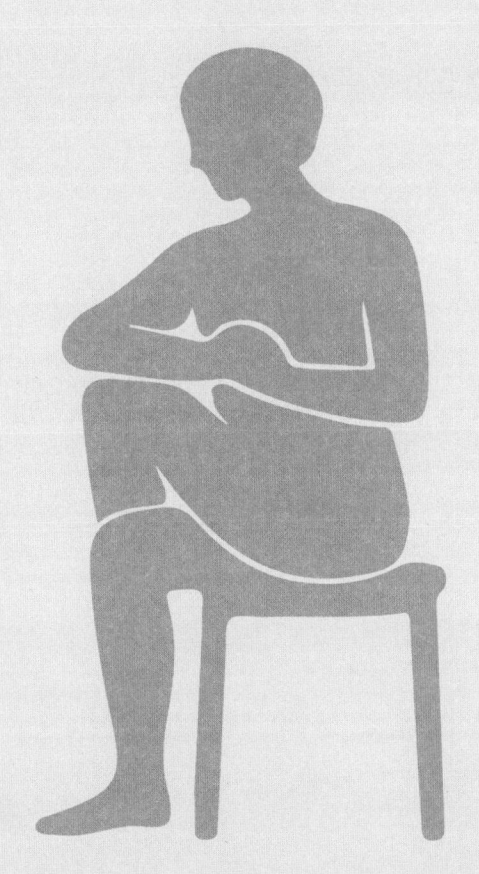

UPPER BODY AND CORE POSES

POSE 23: Seated Single Arm Raise

Type: Shoulder Opener and Spinal Extension
Main Focus: Shoulders, upper back
Secondary Focus: Core, spine

Overview: Seated Single Arm Raise is a simple yet effective pose that focuses on improving shoulder mobility and spinal extension. It helps to open the chest, activate the core, and lengthen the spine, making it a great pose for improving shoulder mobility and relieving tension in the upper body.

Instructions:

1. Sit tall with your feet hip-width apart, engaging your core.
2. Inhale and reach one arm up in front of you until it is in line with your shoulder and parallel with the ground. Keep your arm straight and your palm facing downward.
3. Lengthen through the spine and gently release your shoulders down and back.
4. Hold for several breaths, then slowly release your arm back to your side and repeat on the other side.

Tip:
Avoid arching your lower back as you lift your arm. Keep your core engaged to support a stable, upright posture while lengthening through your spine.

Modifications:
For a more accessible stretch, lift your arm only to the degree at which it feels challenging but not uncomfortable.

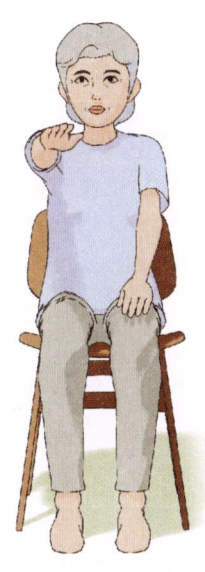
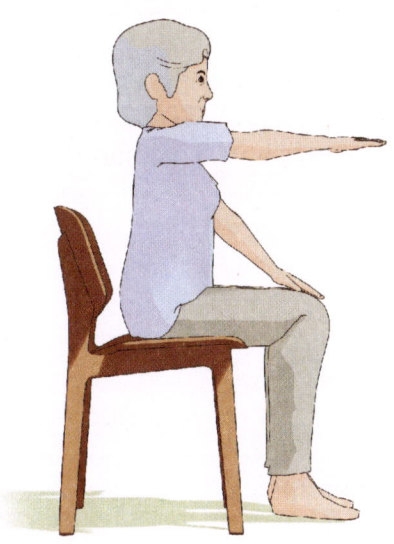

Add-On 1: Single Arm Raise with Wrist Roll
Keep your arm extended in front of you and begin to gently rotate your wrist in a circular motion, moving it clockwise for a few breaths and then reverse the direction for a few breaths.

Add-On 2: Single Arm Raise with Flex and Point
Extend your arm and gently flex your wrist, bending your fingers up toward your forearm. Hold briefly, then slowly point your fingers away to stretch your wrist and forearm. Alternate between flexing and pointing for several breaths.

Add-On 3: Single Arm Raise with Arm Circles
Keep your arm extended out in front of you and begin to rotate your entire arm in small circular motions, moving it clockwise for a few breaths and then reverse the direction for a few breaths.

POSE 24: Seated Yogi Bicep Curls (Single or Double Arm)

Type: Arm Strengthening and Shoulder Mobility
Main Focus: Biceps, shoulders
Secondary Focus: Core, upper back

Overview: Seated Bicep Curls strengthen the arms and biceps while enhancing shoulder mobility. This pose also engages the core for stability, making it a great exercise for building upper body strength and improving shoulder flexibility.

Instructions:

1. Sit tall with your feet hip-width apart, engaging your core.
2. Raise your right arm to shoulder height, with your palm up, and make a fist with your hand. Inhale, then exhale and bend your elbow, bringing your fist toward your shoulder in a controlled motion, activating your biceps.
3. Inhale again, extending your arm back to the starting position and keeping your shoulders relaxed.
4. Repeat for several rounds, moving smoothly between the curl and extension. Repeat on the other side.

Tip:
Focus on slow, controlled movements to fully activate the biceps. Keep your core engaged to support a stable posture and avoid rounding your back.

Modifications:
Reach your arms up only to the degree at which you feel challenged but not uncomfortable. To increase the challenge, hold small weights or bands in your hands while performing the curls.

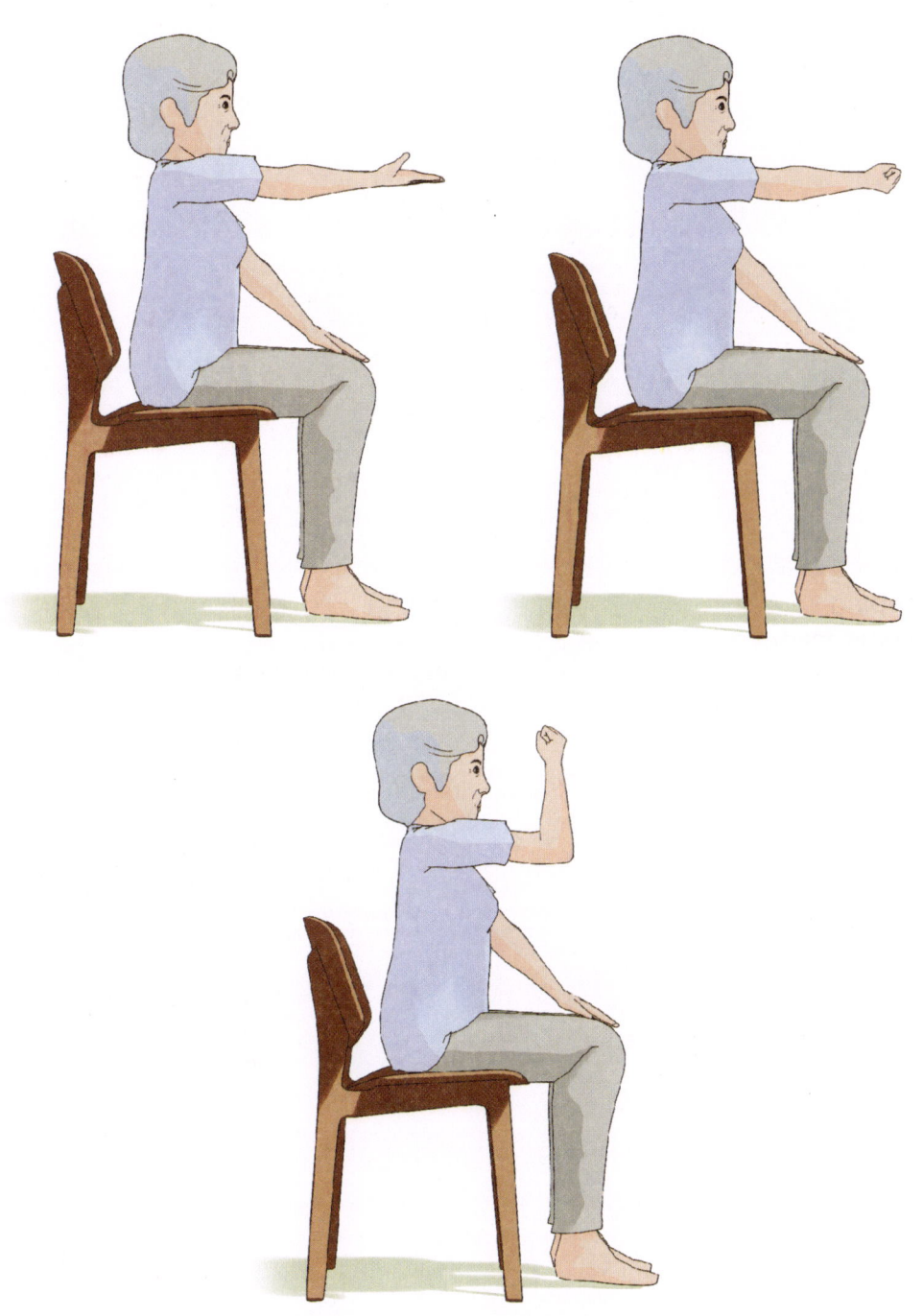

POSE 25: Seated Double Arm Frontal Raise to T Arms

Type: Shoulder Strengthening and Mobility
Main Focus: Shoulders, upper back
Secondary Focus: Core, arms

Overview: Seated Double Arm Frontal Raise to T Arms is a two-part dynamic pose that strengthens the shoulders, arms, and upper back while promoting mobility and stability. It opens the chest and activates the core, helping to improve shoulder flexibility, posture, and overall upper body strength.

Instructions:

1. Inhale and raise both arms in front of you, keeping them straight and parallel to the ground, palms facing downward.
2. As you exhale, move your arms out to the sides, forming a "T" shape with your body.
3. Inhale again and return arms to the front.
4. As you exhale, lower your arms back to your sides.
5. Repeat for several rounds, maintaining smooth, controlled movements throughout.

Tip:
Engage your core throughout the movement to avoid arching your lower back and maintain a strong, stable posture.

Modifications:
For a more accessible stretch, reduce the range of motion, lifting your arms only as high as feels comfortable.

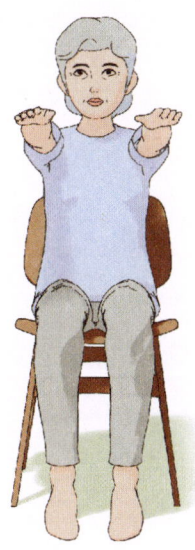
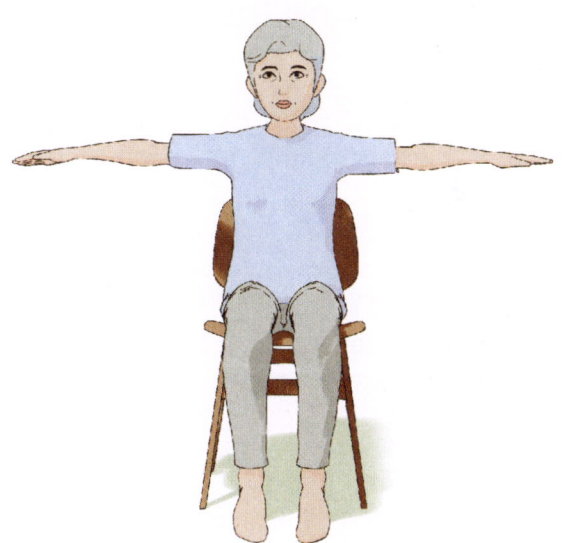

Add-On 1: Micro Arm Circles
After reaching arms to the "T" position, make small circles with your arms, moving in a clockwise direction for several breaths, then reverse the direction for several breaths.

Add-On 2: Palm Flips
While holding the "T" position, inhale and slowly rotate your palms to face upward, then exhale and rotate them back to face downward. Continue flipping your palms for several breaths, focusing on fluid and controlled movements.

POSE 26: Three-Way Seated Wrist Stretch

Type: Wrist Flexibility and Mobility
Main Focus: Wrists, forearms
Secondary Focus: Hands, fingers, arms

Overview: This wrist stretch targets the flexibility and mobility of the wrists, forearms, hands, and fingers. By stretching in different directions, it helps to relieve tension, improve wrist mobility, and prevent strain. It's especially beneficial for those who use their hands and wrists frequently throughout the day.

Instructions:

1. Extend one arm out in front of you, parallel to the ground, with your palm facing downward.
2. Inhale, then as you exhale, use your other hand to pull your fingers back toward your forearm.
3. Hold, then release.
4. Exhale and stretch your wrist in the opposite direction by applying gentle pressure to the back of your hand.
5. Flip your palm up, and push your fingers downward.

Tip:
Move slowly and gently into each stretch, taking a few breaths in each variation. Avoid any jerky movements that could cause strain.

Modifications:
If the stretch feels too intense, reduce the range of motion and focus on gradually deepening the stretch over time. You can also support your wrist with your opposite hand for extra control.

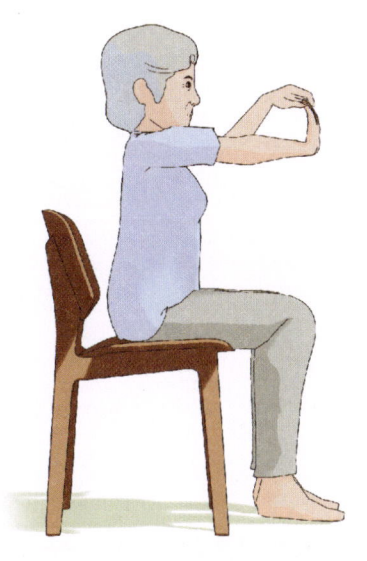

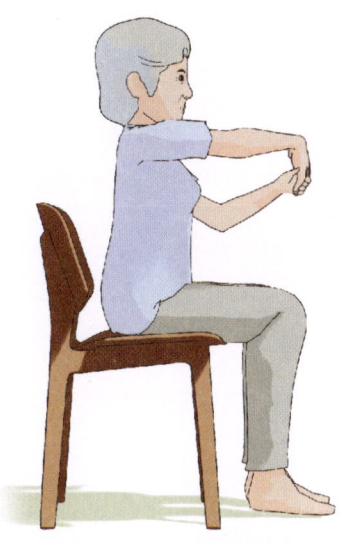

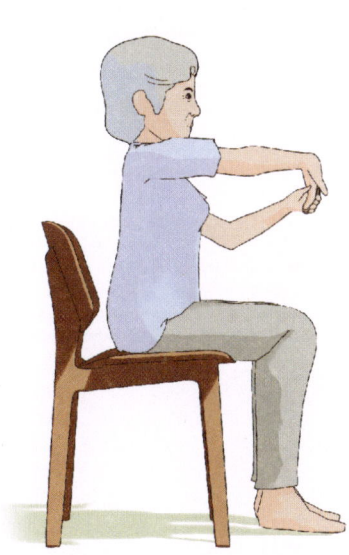

POSE 27: Seated Eagle Arms (Shoulder Grab)

Type: Shoulder Opener and Upper Back Stretch
Main Focus: Shoulders, upper back, lymphatic system
Secondary Focus: Arms, chest, spine

Overview: This pose targets the shoulders and upper back while promoting flexibility in the arms and chest. It helps improve posture, release shoulder tension, and open the upper body, making it ideal for those who spend long hours sitting at a desk. Additionally the pose encourages the movement of lymph fluid, which aids in detoxifying the body and supporting the lymphatic system. By compressing and stretching the arms and shoulders, Seated Eagle Arms promotes improved circulation and helps in the natural detox process.

Instructions:

1. With your arms straight out in front of you, cross your right arm under your left, bringing your forearms perpendicular to the ground.
2. Wrap your forearms around each other and bring your palms to touch.
3. Inhale and lift your elbows toward the ceiling.
4. As you exhale, gently press your hands away from your face.
5. Hold for several breaths.

Tip:
Avoid rounding your back as you lift your elbows. Keep your core engaged and sit tall to maintain proper alignment while deepening the stretch.

Modifications:
If your palms don't reach, use a strap or hold your shoulders instead. For a gentler stretch, keep your arms at a lower height or avoid pressing your palms together.

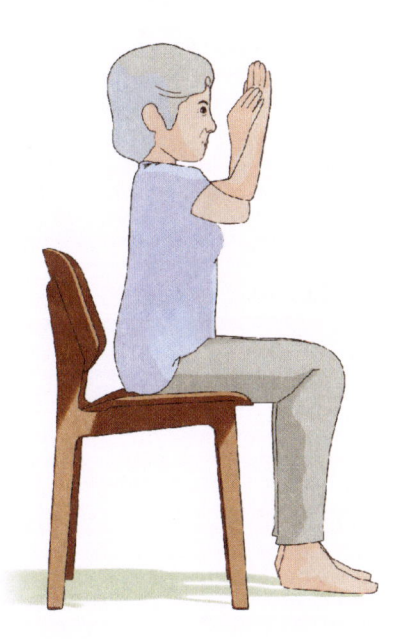
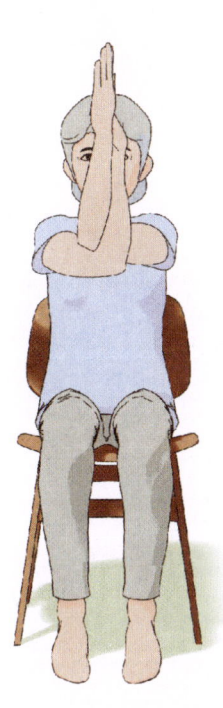

POSE 28: Seated Tricep Stretch

Type: Shoulder and Tricep Stretch
Main Focus: Triceps, shoulders, upper back
Secondary Focus: Arms, chest, lymphatic system

Overview: This pose targets the triceps and shoulders while opening up the chest and improving flexibility. It is beneficial for relieving tension in the arms and shoulders and promoting relaxation. It also encourages lymphatic flow, supporting detoxification and circulation throughout the upper body.

Instructions:

1. Inhale and raise your left arm overhead. Exhale and bend your elbow, bringing your hand down toward your upper back.
2. With your right hand, gently grasp your left elbow and press it toward your head to deepen the stretch.
3. Hold for several breaths, slowly release, and repeat on the other side.

Tip:
Avoid arching your back as you lift your arm. Keep your spine long and engage your core for stability while deepening the stretch.

Modifications:
If your hand doesn't reach your back, just find your fullest expression and gently hold it.

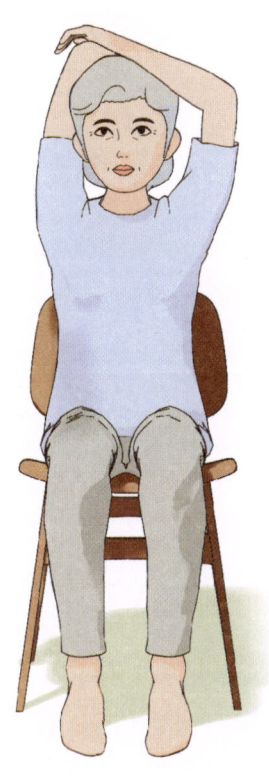

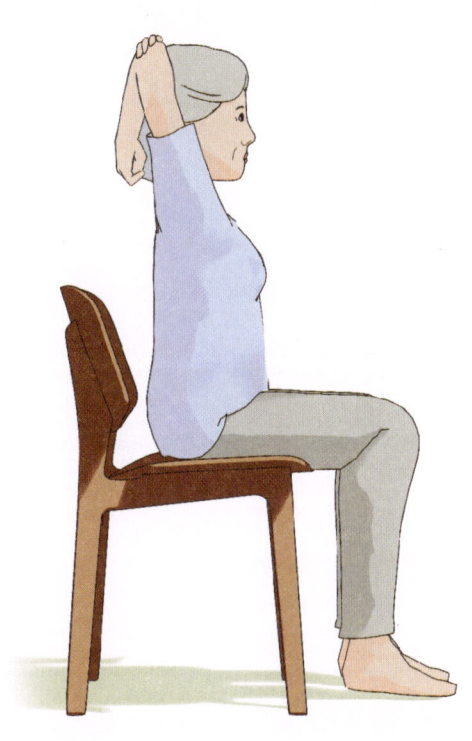

POSE 29: Seated Arm Across Body Shoulder Stretch

Type: Shoulder Opener and Upper Back Stretch
Main Focus: Shoulders, upper back
Secondary Focus: Arms, chest

Overview: This stretch targets the shoulders and upper back while improving flexibility in the arms and chest. This pose helps release tension, improve posture, and open the upper body.

Instructions:

1. Inhale as you extend your right arm straight in front of you at shoulder height and make a fist.
2. As you exhale, bring your right arm across your body at a slight angle, using your right arm to gently pull your left arm closer to your chest.
3. Hold for several breaths, feeling the stretch across your shoulder and upper back.
4. Slowly release and repeat on the other side.

Tip:
Keep your shoulders relaxed as you pull your arm across your body. Avoid rounding your back, and focus on keeping your spine long and your core engaged.

Modifications:
For a gentler stretch, reduce the intensity by not pulling the arm as deeply across the body. If you feel discomfort, avoid using your hand to pull the arm and instead, hold it in place with your own strength.

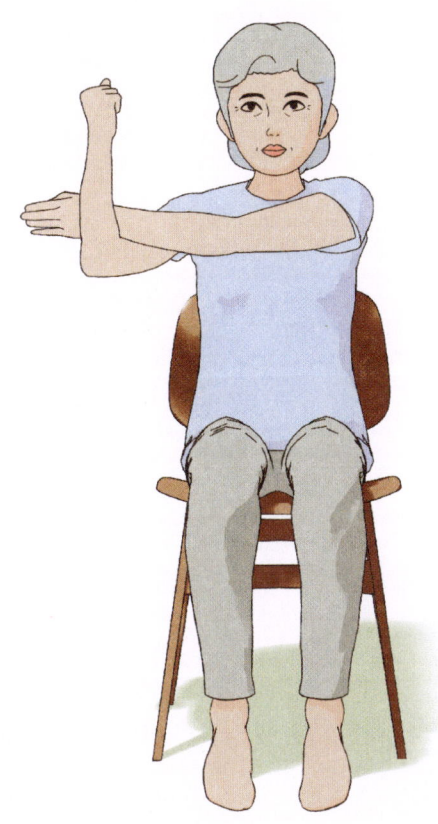

POSE 30: Seated Crunches with Hands Behind Head

Type: Core Activation, Posture Improvement, and Stability
Main Focus: Core, abdominals
Secondary Focus: Lower back, shoulders, lymphatic system

Overview: This is one of the best ways to activate your core and strengthen your abdominals and lower back. This movement stimulates circulation and detoxification from the squeezing and releasing motions, and I love to teach it as a balance stabilizer. It also gets your heart rate up, so it's good for your cardiovascular system. Regular practice enhances spinal alignment, digestion, and body stability, while supporting immune function.

Instructions:

1. Sit tall with your spine straight, your feet flat on the floor, and your hands gently placed behind your head, with your elbows wide.
2. Inhale and slowly open your chest, lifting your upper body toward the sky and pulling your elbows open and back.
3. As you exhale, contract your core, round your spine, and tuck your chin to your chest. Bring your elbows through the center toward your knees.
4. Repeat this movement for several rounds, focusing on the squeeze and release of your core.

Tip:
Avoid pulling on your neck with your hands. The deeper you breathe in this pose, the better it will feel.

Modifications:
Reduce the range of motion or keep your hands at your temples instead of behind your head.

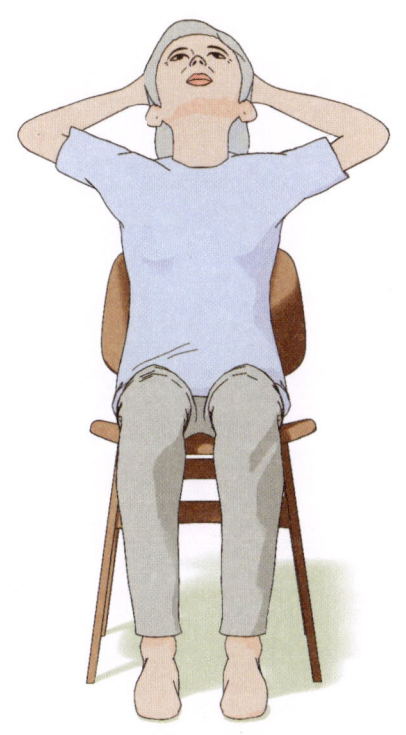

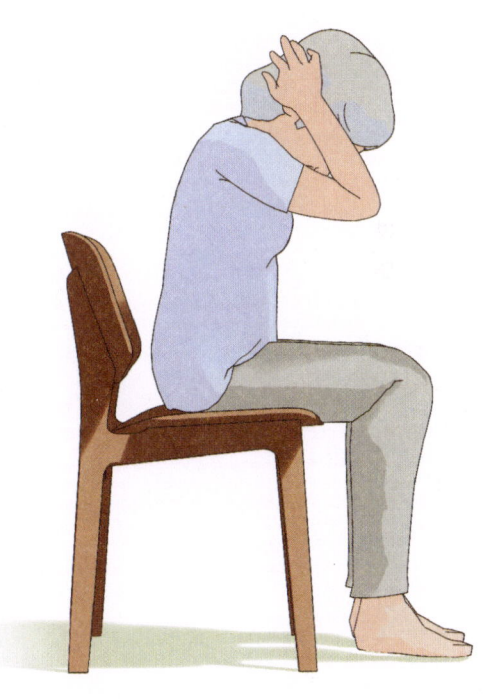

5-MINUTE UPPER BODY RELIEF

These sequences target the neck, shoulders, arms, and upper back—the areas where we hold the most stress. They are ideal for anyone who spends time at a computer, carries tension up high, or needs a quick desk break.

- Desk Break
  - Three-Way Seated Wrist Stretch (2 min)
  - Seated Eagle Arms (1.5 min each side)

- Shoulder Soother
  - Seated Single Arm Raise with Arm Circles (2 min)
  - Seated Tricep Stretch (1.5 min each side)

- Strength Builder
  - Seated Single Arm Raise with Bicep Curls (2 min)
  - Seated Double Arm Frontal Raises to T Arms (3 min)

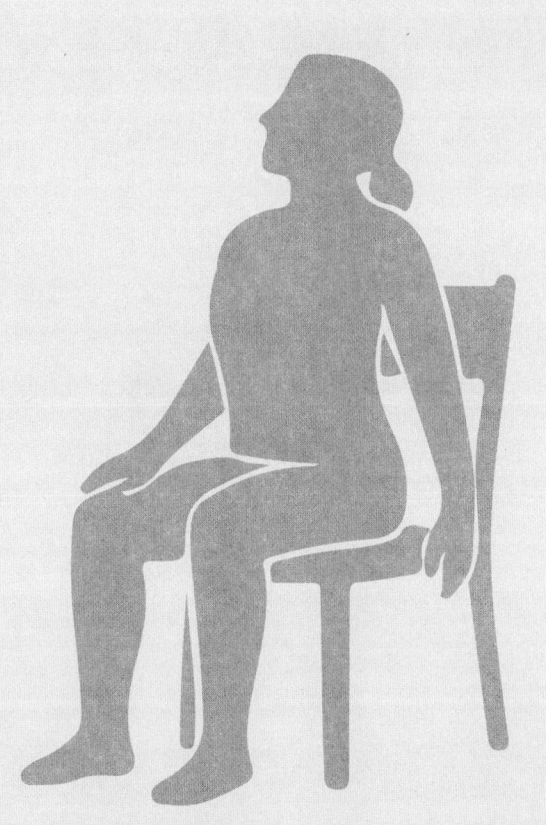

HEAD, NECK, AND SHOULDER POSES

POSE 31: Seated Ear to Shoulder Pose

Type: Neck and Shoulder Stretch
Main Focus: Neck, shoulders, trapezius muscles
Secondary Focus: Upper back

Overview: This stretch is designed to target the neck and shoulders, helping to release tension and improve flexibility. This pose is great for relaxation and can alleviate discomfort caused by tightness in the neck and upper back, especially from sitting for long periods. You can practice this at any time for gentle release in the upper body or to ease tension headaches.

Instructions:

1. Inhale deeply, and as you exhale, gently lower your left ear toward your left shoulder.
2. To deepen the stretch, use your left hand to gently apply pressure to your left temple, encouraging the stretch in your neck and shoulder.
3. Hold for several breaths, feeling the stretch along the side of your neck and across the shoulder.
4. Slowly release the stretch, and repeat it on the opposite side.

Tip:
Keep your spine straight and avoid tilting your head forward. Ensure your shoulders remain relaxed and away from your ears to avoid additional tension.

Modifications:
For a gentler stretch, reduce the range of motion in your neck and don't apply pressure with your hand.

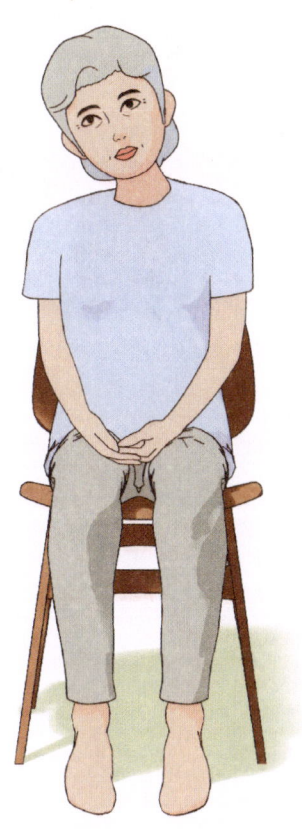
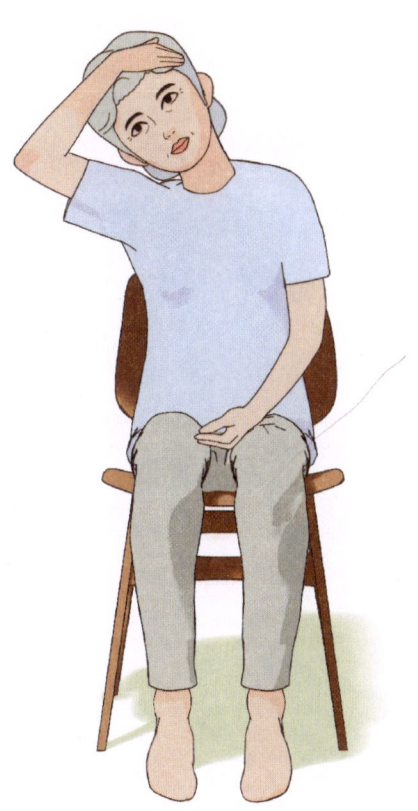

POSE 32: Seated Chin to Chest Pose

Type: Neck and Upper Back Stretch
Main Focus: Neck, upper back
Secondary Focus: Shoulders, spine

Overview: This stretch targets the neck and upper back, helping to alleviate tension and improve flexibility in your cervical spine. It can also promote better posture and relieve discomfort from poor alignment or extended periods of sitting. This is a great stretch for when you first wake up in the morning.

Instructions:

1. Inhale deeply, and as you exhale, gently lower your chin toward your chest, bringing the back of your neck into a stretch.
2. Reaching your hands toward your knees, hold the position, allowing gravity to deepen the stretch.
3. Hold for several breaths, keeping your shoulders relaxed and away from your ears.
4. Slowly raise your chin back up to neutral and return to your starting position.

Tip:
Avoid forcing your chin to your chest. Focus on gently lengthening your neck as you move into the stretch, and maintain a relaxed posture throughout the entire stretch.

Modifications:
For a gentler stretch, don't lower your chin as deeply and keep your hands relaxed in your lap.

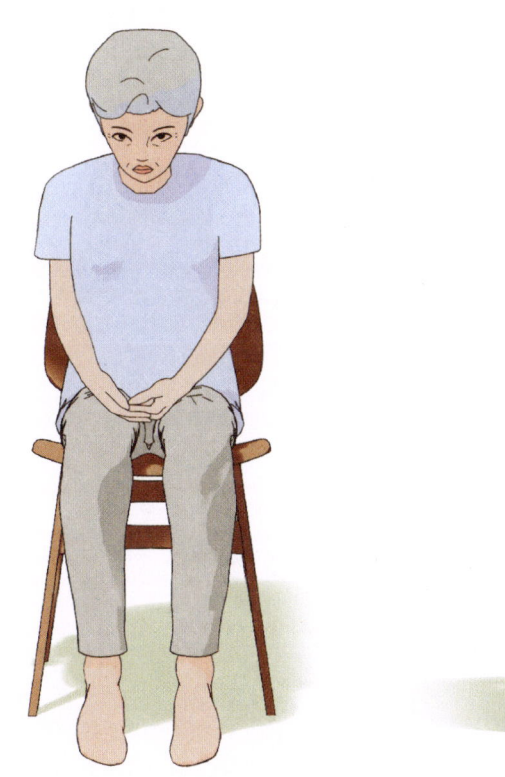
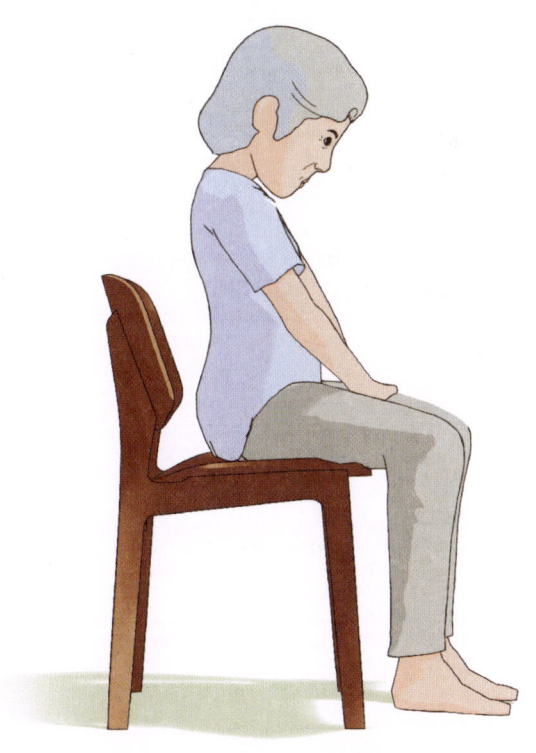

POSE 33: Seated Neck Rolls

Type: Neck and Shoulder Mobility
Main Focus: Neck, shoulders
Secondary Focus: Upper back, trapezius muscles

Overview: Neck rolls help to improve mobility in the neck and shoulders, easing tension. This movement increases circulation, relieves stiffness, and can be particularly helpful for those who spend long periods in front of a screen.

Instructions:

1. Inhale, then exhale. Gently bring your chin toward your chest.
2. Begin to slowly roll your head in a circular motion, allowing your chin to move from your chest to your left shoulder, then up toward the ceiling, around to your right shoulder, and back down toward your chest.
3. Continue the motion, breathing deeply and allowing your neck to move fluidly through the range of motion.
4. Complete several rolls in one direction, then repeat the movements in the opposite direction.

Tip:
Keep your shoulders relaxed and avoid hunching as you roll your neck. Move slowly and mindfully, and don't push your head too far in any direction—let your neck move naturally.

Modifications:
For a gentler version, reduce the size of the circles and avoid any jerky movements.

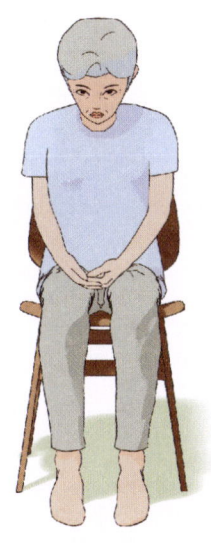
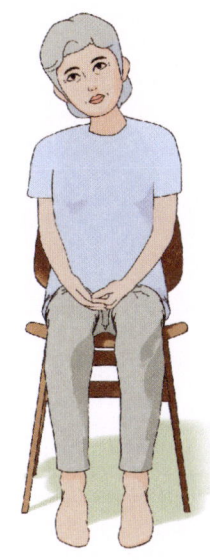
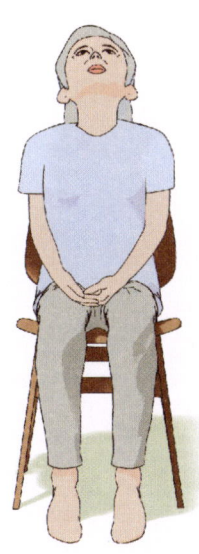
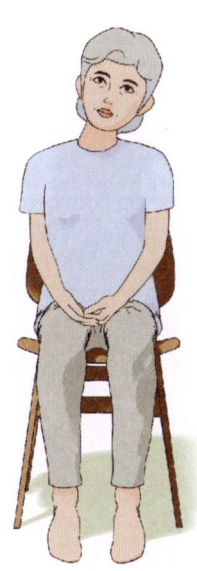

POSE 34: Seated Neck Twists

Type: Neck and Upper Back Range of Motion
Main Focus: Neck, upper back
Secondary Focus: Shoulders, cervical spine

Overview: Neck twists feel amazing and are great for relieving tension built up from sleeping or sitting in one position for extended periods of time. This movement can increase circulation, improve posture, and offer a gentle way to calm your nervous system.

Instructions:

1. Inhale deeply, and as you exhale, gently rotate your head to the left, bringing your chin toward your left shoulder, and look toward the back of the room.
2. Hold the position for a few breaths, then inhale to return to the center.
3. As you exhale, rotate your head to the right, bringing your chin toward your right shoulder.
4. Repeat this twisting motion several times on each side.

Tip:
Keep your shoulders relaxed and avoid forcing your neck into a deep twist. Move gently and listen to your body, making sure to keep your spine tall and aligned throughout.

Modifications:
If you feel discomfort, reduce the range of motion by rotating only slightly to each side. You can also use your hand to gently guide the twist, but avoid applying excessive pressure.

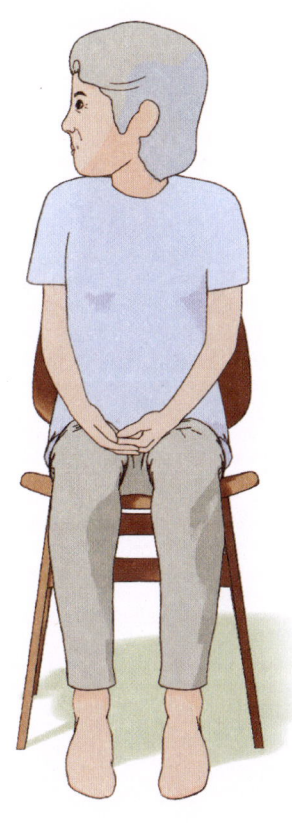 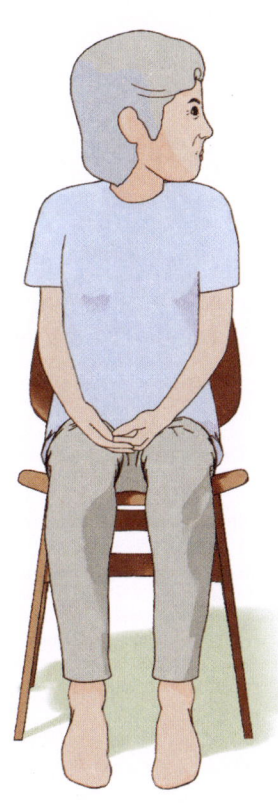

POSE 35: Seated Shoulders to Ears with Drop

Type: Shoulder Mobility, Tension Release, and Lymphatic Stimulation
Main Focus: Shoulders, upper back
Secondary Focus: Neck, arms, lymphatic system

Overview: The Shoulders to Ears with Drop movement helps to release tension in the shoulders and upper back while promoting better shoulder mobility. This movement stimulates the lymphatic system, encouraging circulation and aiding in detoxification by helping to move lymph fluid throughout the body. It's especially beneficial for relieving stress and improving overall circulation.

Instructions:

1. Inhale deeply.
2. As you exhale, lift your shoulders toward your ears, engaging your upper back and neck.
3. Hold briefly, allowing the muscles to contract, then exhale as you release your shoulders, letting them drop down and away from your ears, relaxing completely.
4. Repeat several times, focusing on the contrast between the tension and the release, while feeling the stimulation of your lymphatic flow.

Tip:
Avoid rounding your back or shrugging your shoulders forward as you lift them. Keep your chest open and focus on gently dropping your shoulders down and back, allowing for a full release of tension and smooth circulation.

Modifications:
Move slowly and mindfully, allowing the muscles to gradually release and flow freely.

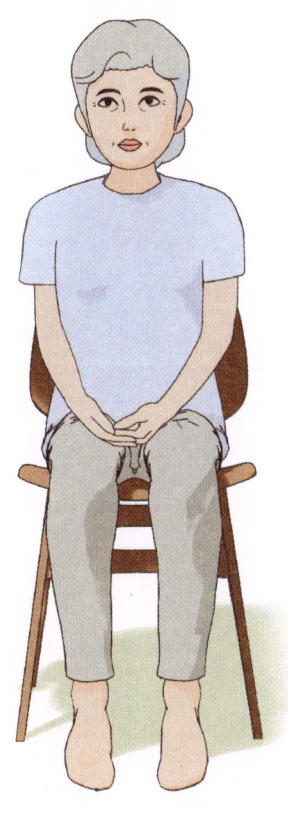
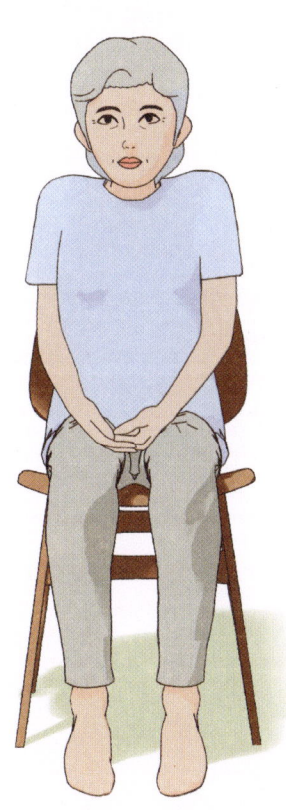

POSE 36: Seated Shoulder Rolls

Type: Shoulder Mobility, Tension Relief, Lymphatic Stimulation, and Nervous System Calming
Main Focus: Shoulders, upper back
Secondary Focus: Neck, arms, lymphatic system, nervous system

Overview: Shoulder rolls calm the nervous system, helping to release pressure and tension while improving shoulder mobility. This movement stimulates the lymphatic system by encouraging fluid circulation, aiding detoxification, and enhancing overall circulation. Regular practice promotes relaxation, reduces stress, and supports lymphatic drainage, which is essential for maintaining a healthy immune system.

Instructions:

1. Inhale deeply and gently roll your shoulders forward in a circular motion.
2. As you exhale, continue the rolling motion, completing a few circles, then reverse direction, rolling your shoulders back and down.
3. Focus on smooth, controlled movements, allowing your muscles to relax and release any built-up tension.

Tip:
Keep your movements slow and mindful. Engage your core to support your spine while focusing on releasing tension with each roll.

Modifications:
Move gently and slowly, and reduce the range of motion if needed.

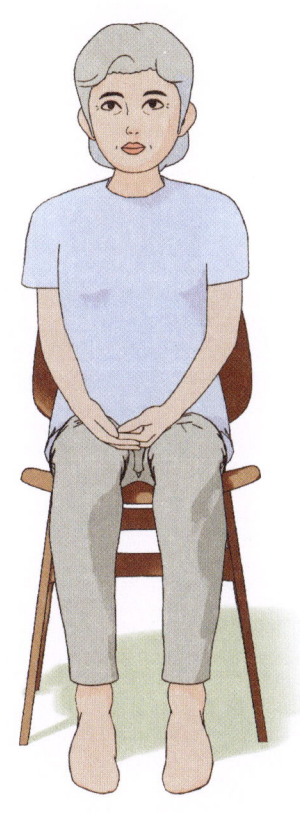
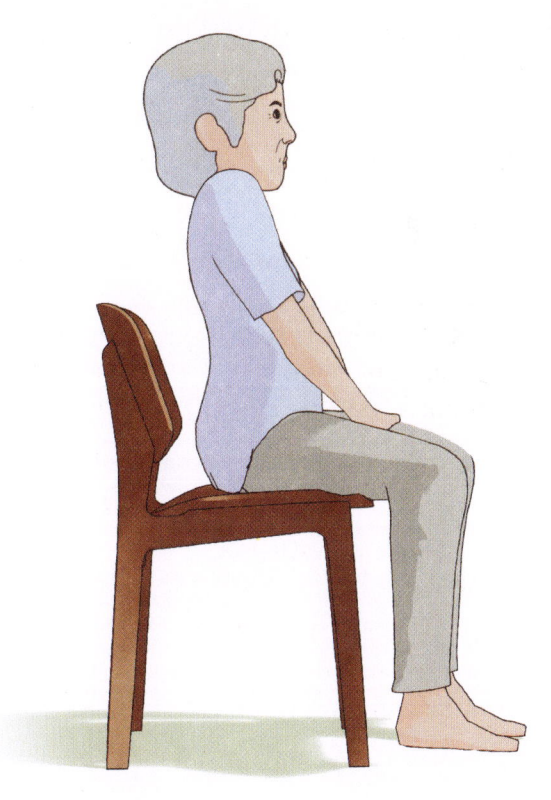

5-MINUTE TENSION TAMERS

When stress shows up in your body as tightness and discomfort, these gentle combinations offer sweet relief. Focus on the areas where you personally hold tension—your body will thank you.

- Neck Relief
  - Seated Ear to Shoulder Pose (1 min each side)
  - Seated Neck Rolls (2 min

- Shoulder Reset
  - Seated Shoulder Rolls (2 min)
  - Seated Shoulders to Ears with Drop (1 min)
  - Seated Neck Twists (2 min)

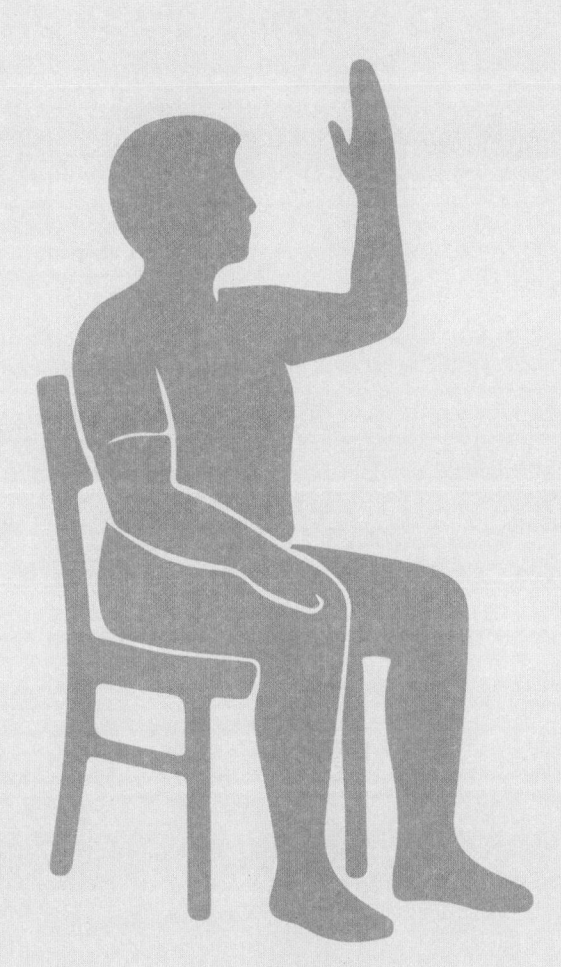

SUPPORTED STANDING POSES (ADVANCED)

Important Note: These standing poses are optional and more advanced. Only practice these if you can comfortably rise from your chair and stand steadily without additional support. They're perfect for building toward greater independence, strength, and balance.

POSE 37: Supported Standing One-Legged Balance (*Tadasana*)

Type: Balance and Stability
Main Focus: Core, legs, balance
Secondary Focus: Hips, ankles

Overview: Tadasana improves balance and stability by strengthening the core and legs. Regular practice enhances posture, strengthens the lower body, and improves coordination.

Instructions:

1. Stand tall with your hands holding the back of your chair and your feet hip-width apart, engaging your core for stability.
2. Shift your weight onto your right leg, lift your left leg, and bend your knee at 90 degrees, keeping your foot flexed.
3. Hold for several breaths, slowly release, then repeat on the other side.

Tip:
Keep your gaze focused on a fixed point to help with balance. Engage your core to support your spine and avoid letting your hips drop out of alignment or arching your lower back.

Modifications:
If you struggle with balance, try sitting on your chair instead.

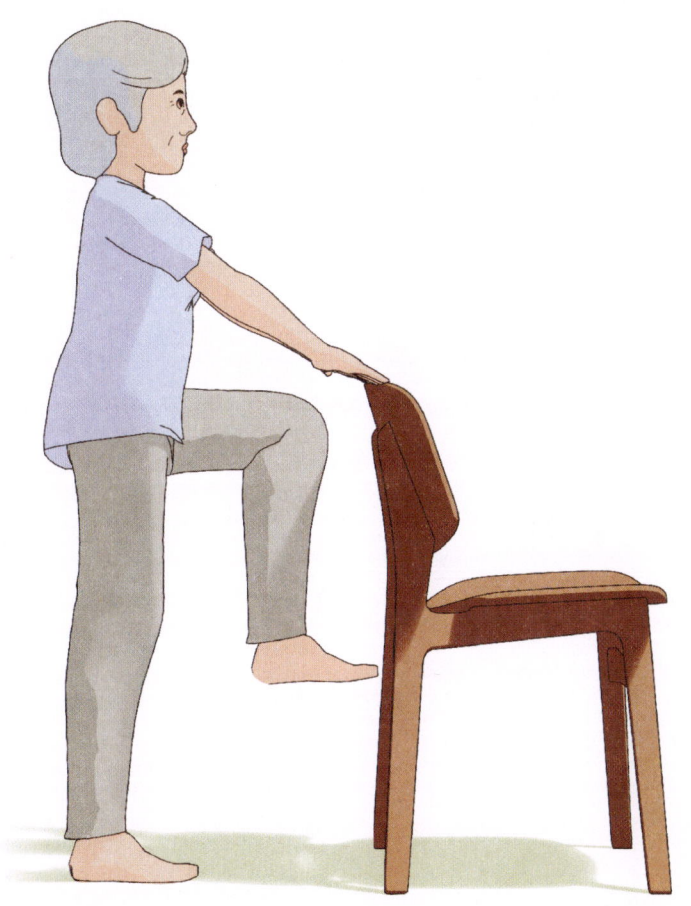

POSE 38: Supported Standing Downward Facing Dog

Type: Full Body Stretch, Flexibility, and Balance
Main Focus: Hamstrings, calves, shoulders
Secondary Focus: Spine, hips, lymphatic system

Overview: This balancing posture stretches the hamstrings, calves, and shoulders while opening the hips and spine. It is a great posture to test your balance and stability and is wonderful for circulation as it brings your heart in line with your hips, creating a slight inversion.

Instructions:

1. Stand facing a sturdy chair with your feet hip-width apart. Place your hands on the back of the chair, keeping your arms straight.
2. Inhale, and as you exhale, take a big step back with each foot. Hinge at your hips, lifting your hips toward the ceiling, forming an inverted "V" shape.
3. Keep your gaze down and your spine long, and stretch your hamstrings and calves, ensuring your head and neck stay aligned with your spine.
4. Hold for several breaths, focusing on deep breathing and stretching.

Tip:
Engage your core to support your lower back. Keep your legs straight but not locked, allowing for a gentle stretch in your hamstrings.

Modifications:
For a gentler stretch, bend your knees slightly to reduce the strain on your hamstrings.

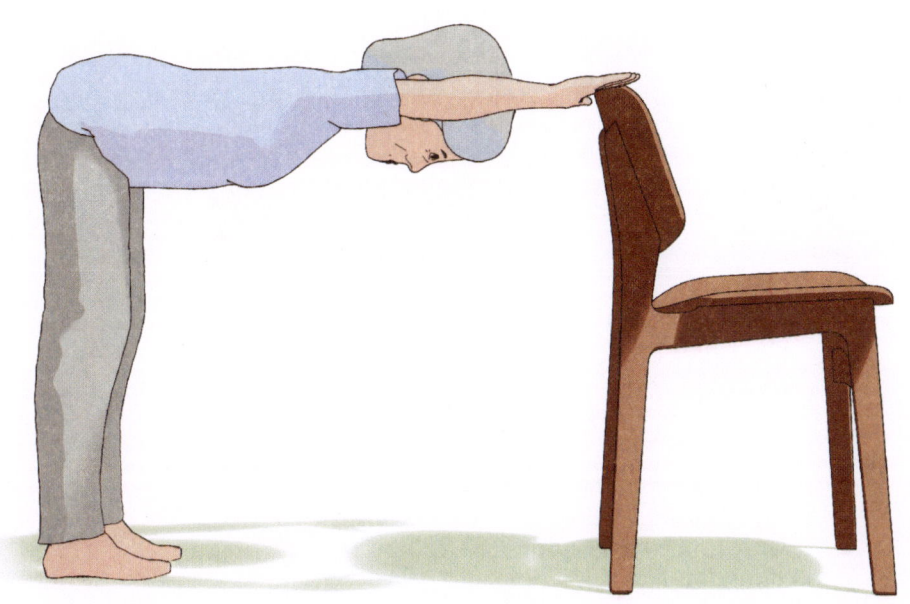

POSE 39: Supported Balancing Warrior Three

Type: Balance, Core Activation, and Leg Strengthening
Main Focus: Core, legs, balance
Secondary Focus: Hips, spine, arms

Overview: Supported Balancing Warrior Three strengthens the core and legs while challenging your balance, concentration, and stability. Using a chair, this pose helps to activate the core, engages the legs, and opens the hips.

Instructions:

1. Stand tall and place your hands on the back of the chair for support, engaging your core.
2. Inhale, then exhale as you shift your weight onto your right leg, lifting your left leg behind you.
3. Keeping your right leg straight and your hips level, reach your torso forward, creating a straight line from your head to your heel.
4. Hold for several breaths, then gently return to standing and repeat on the other side.

Tip:
Focus your gaze on a fixed point in front of you to help with stability.

Modifications:
For more support, just come onto the toes of the foot you are lifting instead of lifting it all the way.

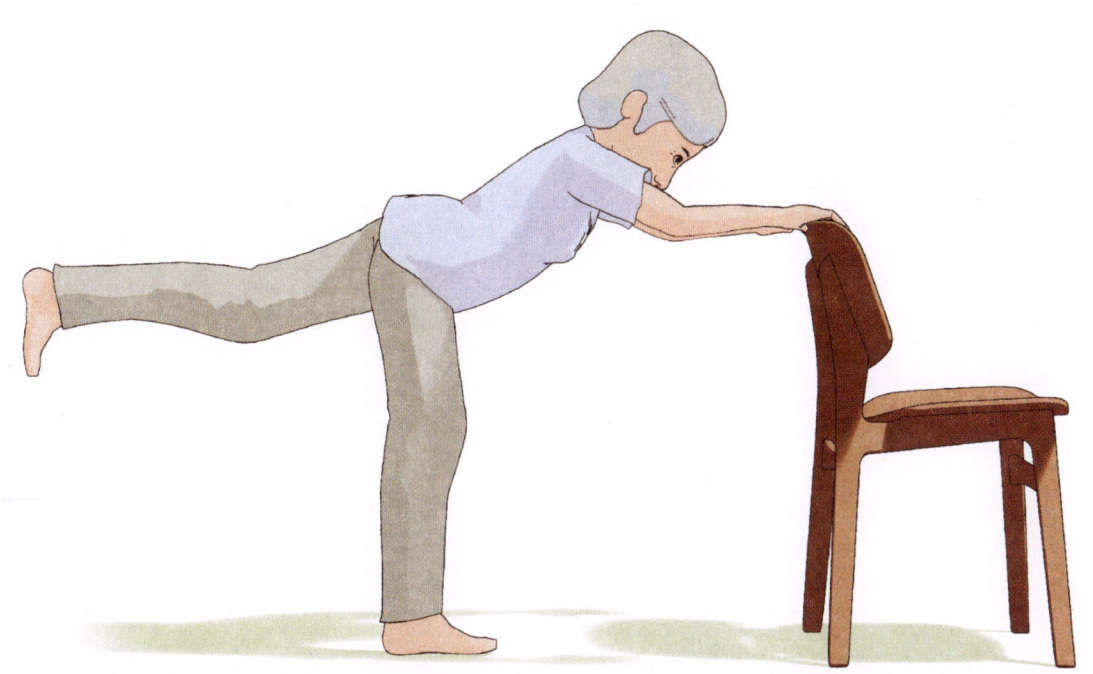

POSE 40: Supported Balancing Tree Pose

Type: Balance, Leg Strengthening, and Hip Opening
Main Focus: Legs, hips, balance
Secondary Focus: Core, spine, arms

Overview: This pose is a hip opener that also challenges your balance and focus. While standing strong in this shape, you also boost your confidence by broadening your chest. Using a chair for support makes it accessible while still offering a deep stretch for the legs and hips, enhancing overall body stability.

Instructions:

1. Stand tall behind your chair with your feet hip-width apart. Place your right hand on the back of the chair for support and engage your core.
2. Inhale, then exhale as you lift your left foot to your inner right thigh or calf (avoiding the knee).
3. Keep your hand on the chair in front of you for support. Hold for several breaths, and then repeat it on the other side.

Tip:
Focus on a fixed point in front of you to maintain balance. Keep your standing leg slightly bent for added stability, and engage your core throughout.

Modifications:
If balancing is challenging, keep your lifted foot lower, rest it against your ankle, or keep your toes on the ground.

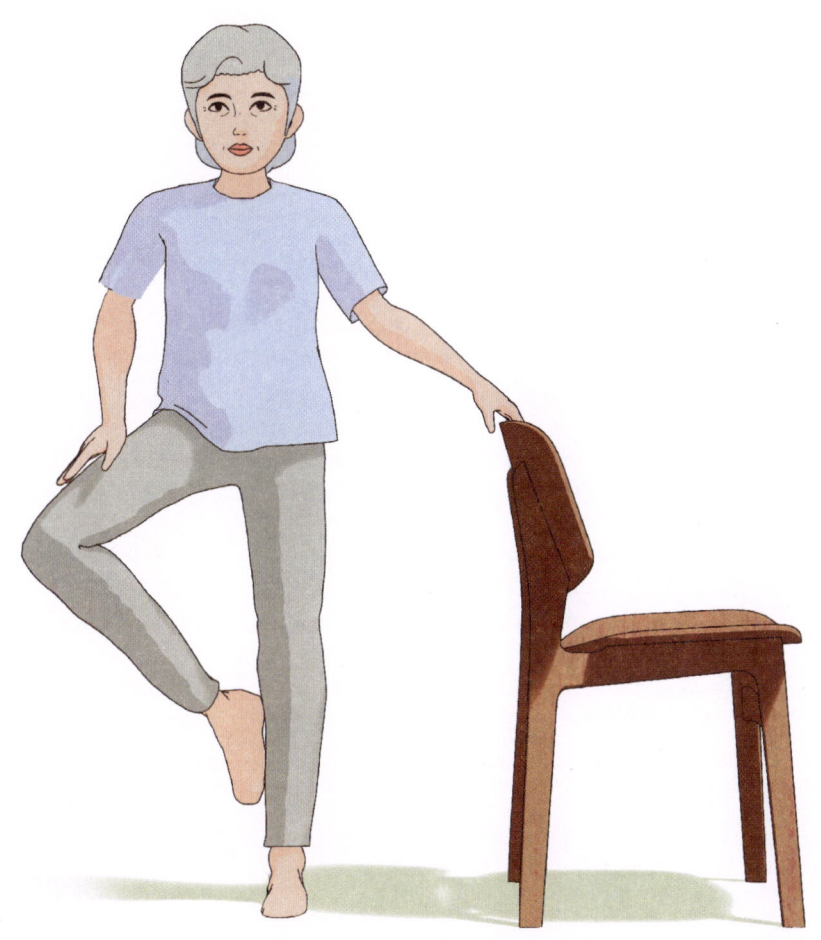

POSE 41: Supported Standing Heel Raises

Type: Leg Strengthening and Balance
Main Focus: Legs, calves, balance
Secondary Focus: Core, ankles

Overview: Supported Standing Heel Raises strengthen your calves and improve the balance that is needed for walking. Using a chair for support makes the pose accessible, allowing you to build strength and confidence without straining, and improves overall lower body strength and circulation.

Instructions:

1. Stand tall behind your chair with your feet hip-width apart. Place your hands on the back of the chair for support, and engage your core.
2. Inhale, then exhale as you slowly lift your heels off the ground, rising onto the balls of your feet.
3. Hold for a few breaths, then slowly lower your heels back to the floor.
4. Repeat for several rounds, focusing on controlled movement.

Tip:
Keep your core engaged, and avoid leaning forward. Focus on rising smoothly, using your legs and calves to lift yourself, not just your ankles.

Modifications:
If balancing is challenging, perform the exercise with less height. If needed, take breaks between repetitions.

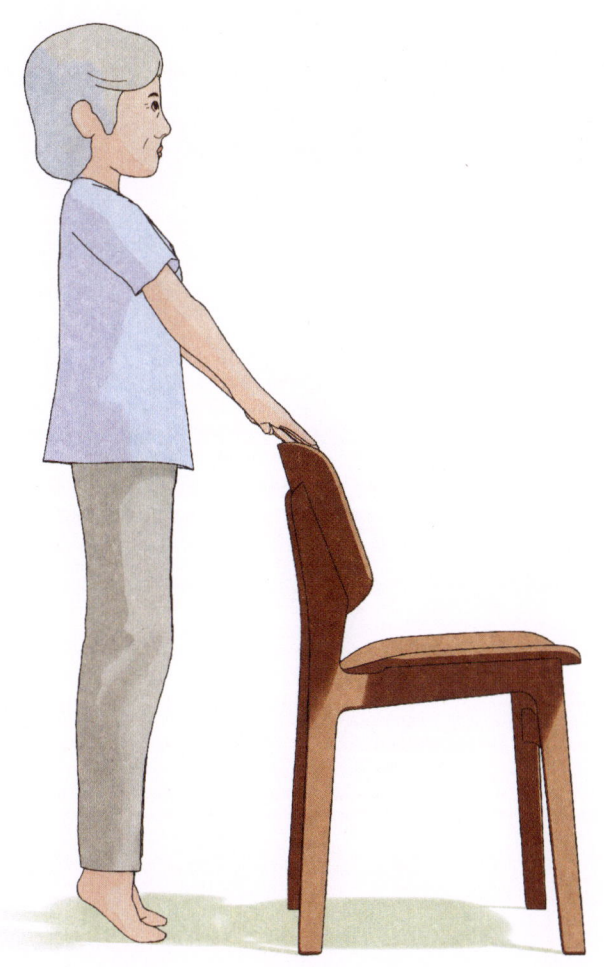

POSE 42: Supported Standing Chair Pose

Type: Leg Strengthening, Core Activation, and Posture Improvement
Main Focus: Legs, core
Secondary Focus: Hips, spine, arms

Overview: Supported Standing Chair Pose strengthens the legs and core and improves posture while enhancing balance. By using a chair for support, you can focus on building strength in the lower body without overstraining, helping to improve flexibility and stability, and engaging the muscles of the hips, thighs, and abdomen.

Instructions:

1. Stand tall behind your chair with your feet hip-width apart. Place your hands on the back of the chair for support, and engage your core.
2. Inhale, and as you exhale, bend your knees, lowering your hips as if sitting into an imaginary chair.
3. Keep your chest lifted, your spine long, and your knees tracking over your toes. Hold the pose for several breaths, then slowly rise back up to standing.

Tip:
Keep your weight in your heels, and avoid letting your knees pass too far over your toes. Focus on keeping your back straight and engaging your core to protect your lower back.

Modifications:
If you need extra support, reduce the depth of your squat.

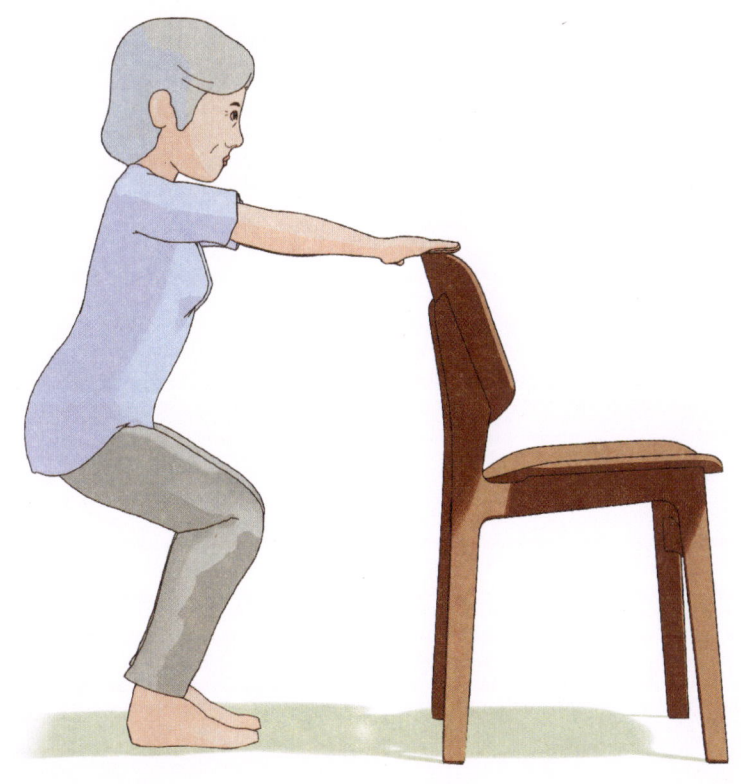

Add-On 1: Chair Squats
Repeat lifting and lowering into your squat for several rounds, maintaining a strong core and steady breath throughout.

POSE 43: Supported Standing Crescent Warrior

Type: Leg Strengthening, Balance, and Hip Flexion
Main Focus: Legs, hips, core
Secondary Focus: Arms, shoulders, spine

Overview: Supported Standing Crescent Warrior is a balancing pose that strengthens the legs, hips, and core while improving balance and flexibility. This pose also helps open the hips and stretches the thighs, enhancing stability and overall body strength. It's a powerful pose!

Instructions:

1. Stand tall behind your chair with your feet hip-width apart. Place your hands on the back of the chair for support and engage your core.
2. Step your right foot back, keeping your left knee bent and aligned over your left ankle.
3. Inhale, and as you exhale, lower your hips, keeping your hands on the chair, your chest open, and your back leg straight.
4. Challenge yourself by lifting your back heel up off the mat.

Tip:
Ensure that your back leg is straight and strong, and avoid letting your front knee extend past your toes.

Modifications:
If you need more support, reduce the depth of your lunge.

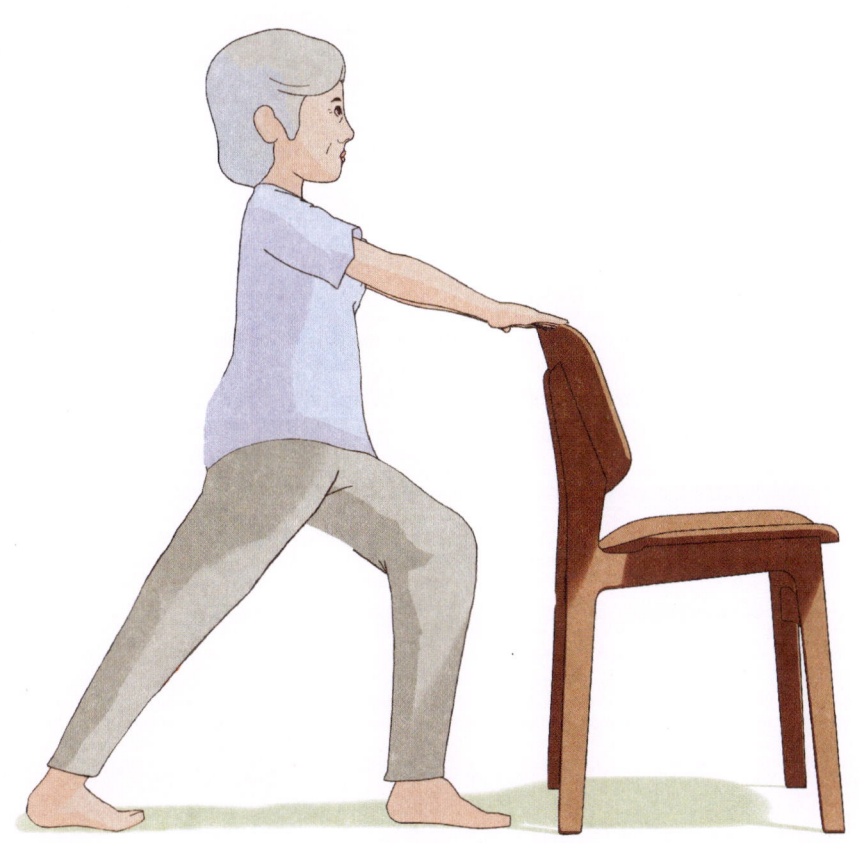

POSE 44: Supported Standing Warrior Two

Type: Leg Strengthening, Balance, and Hip Opener
Main Focus: Legs, hips, arms
Secondary Focus: Core, shoulders, spine

Overview:

Supported Standing Warrior Two is the pose of a warrior: strong, fierce, and a courageous stance of transformation. It also strengthens the legs, hips, and arms while promoting balance and stability.

Instructions1.

1. Stand tall behind your chair with your feet hip-width apart. Place your hands on the back of the chair for support, and engage your core.
2. Take a big step back with your left leg and turn the left foot 90 degrees. Bend your right knee, keeping it aligned over your ankle.
3. Open your shoulders and hips so that they face the left side of the room, and for an added challenge, reach your right arm behind you.
4. Hold the position for several breaths, then slowly return to the center and repeat it on the other side.

Tip:

Keep your shoulders relaxed and your chest open. Ensure your front knee is tracking over your toes, and engage your core to support your spine.

Modifications:

If balance is challenging, reduce the depth of the lunge and keep both hands on the chair.

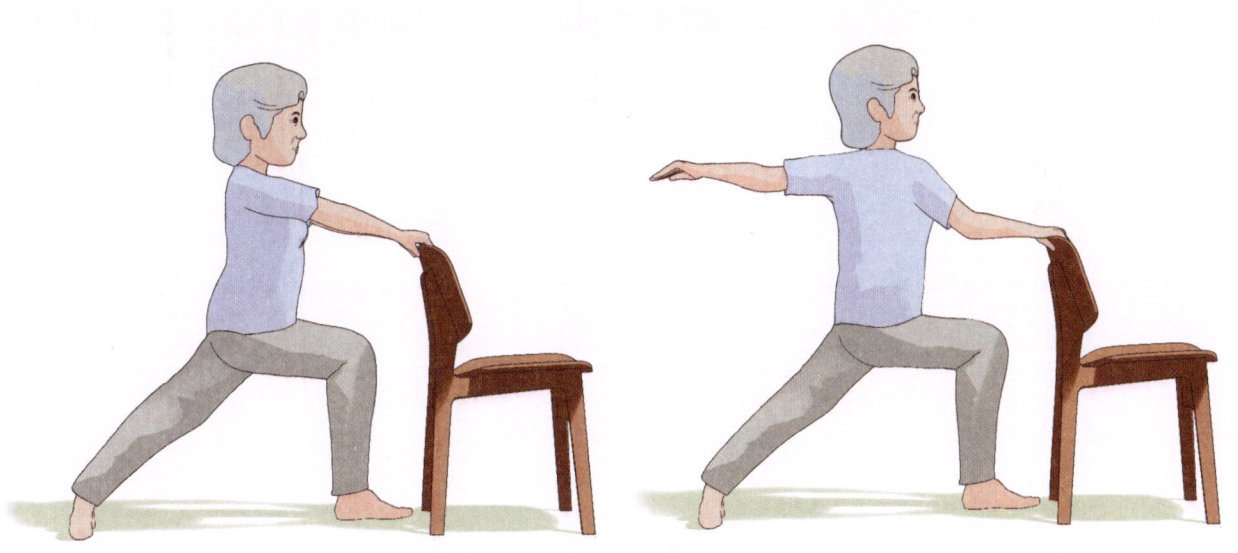

POSE 45: Supported Standing Pyramid Pose

Type: Hamstring Stretch, Leg Strengthening, and Balance
Main Focus: Hamstrings, legs, core
Secondary Focus: Hips, spine, shoulders

Overview: Supported Standing Pyramid Pose stretches the hamstrings and strengthens the legs while promoting balance, stability, and focus. This pose feels great if you have tight legs and hips, and it is often considered a more advanced posture.

Instructions:

1. Stand tall behind your chair with your feet hip-width apart. Place your hands on the back of the chair for support, and engage your core.
2. Step your right foot back about 3–4 feet, keeping your feet parallel, your hips squared, and your back heel on the floor.
3. With your hands on the chair, slowly hinge forward at the hips, lowering your torso toward your right leg.
4. Keep your right leg straight to stretch your hamstrings, and maintain a long spine.
5. Hold for several breaths, then return to standing and repeat on the other side.

Tip:
Keep your hips squared and engage your core to protect your lower back. Avoid rounding your back, and focus on lengthening through your spine as you fold forward.

Modifications:
For a gentler stretch, use a higher chair for support or keep a slight bend in your front knee. Reduce the depth of the stretch as needed to maintain comfort.

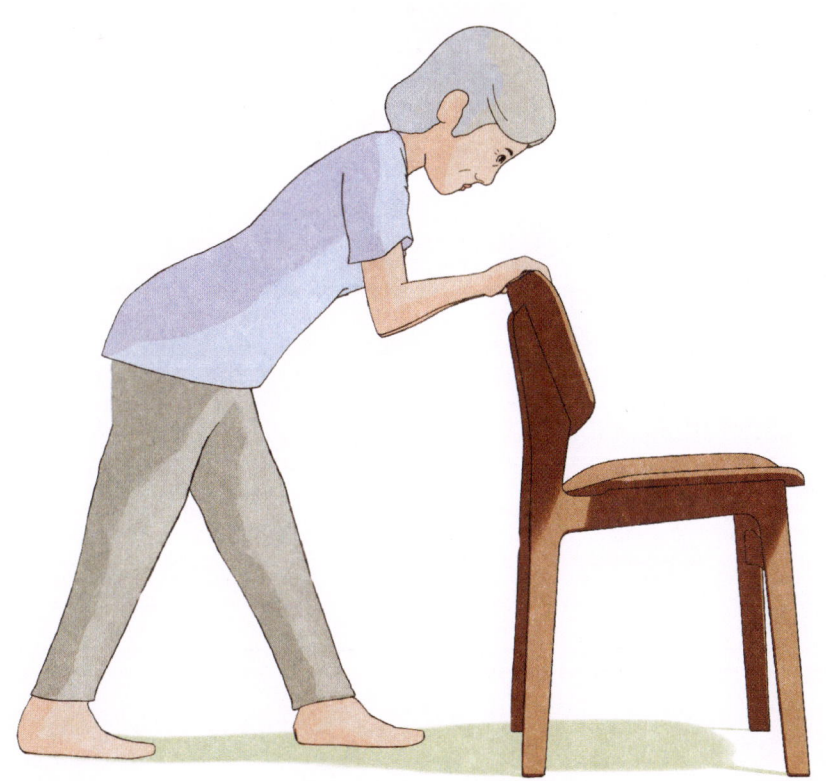

5-MINUTE STANDING CHALLENGES

Ready to test your balance and build strength? These standing sequences use your chair for support while challenging your body in new ways. Perfect for days when you're feeling strong and adventurous.

- Balance Builder
  - Supported Balancing Tree Pose (2 min each side)
  - Supported Standing Heel Raises (1 min)

- Strength Session
  - Chair Squats (2 min)
  - Supported Standing Warrior Two (3 min)

- Gentle Standing
  - Seated Extended Mountain (2 min)
  - Supported Pyramid Pose (3 min)

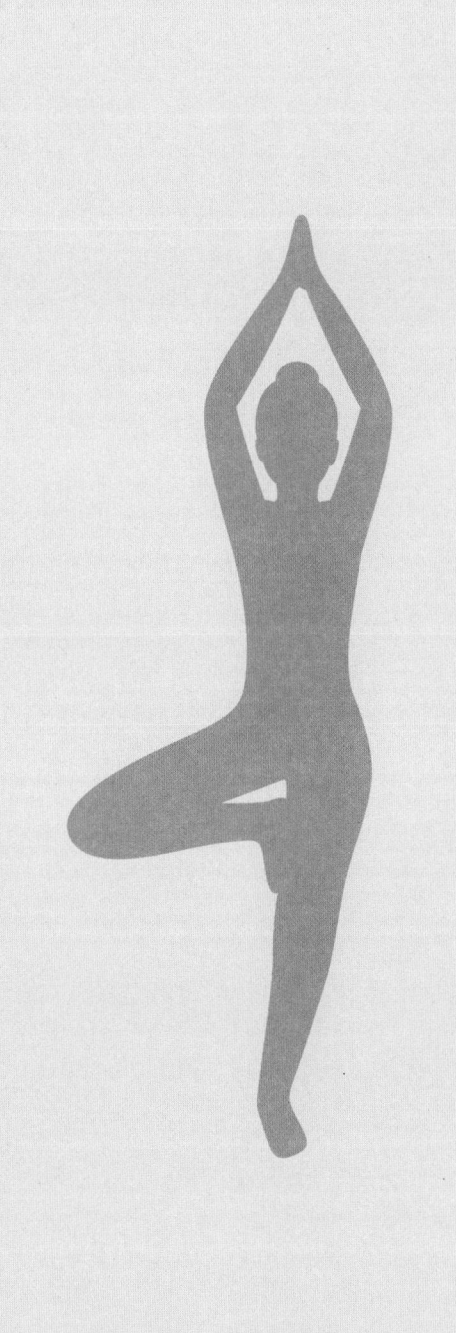

PART 3

YOUR 5-MINUTE SEQUENCES

Welcome to your ready-made 5-minute practices! This section contains nine complete sequences, each designed to fit perfectly into five minutes. Whether you need to wake up your spine, strengthen your core, or find some calm, there's a sequence here for you.

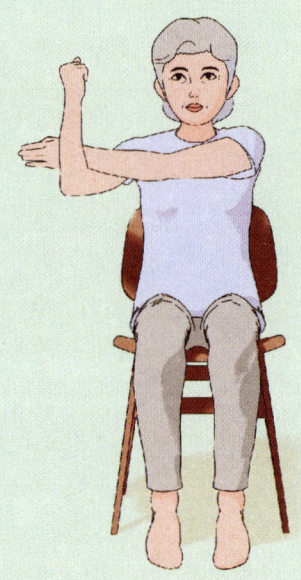

How to Use These Sequences

Each sequence is:

- Timed to five minutes with suggested breath counts and hold times
- Complete on its own—no need to add anything
- Focused on a specific goal—choose based on what you need
- Adaptable—modify any pose to suit your body

Your 5-Minute Practice Menu

1. **CAT-COW FLOW:** gentle spine awakening
2. **SUN SALUTATION A:** energizing full-body warm-up
3. **SUN SALUTATION–WARRIOR FLOW:** warrior flow for strength
4. **HIP MOBILITY MAGIC:** release lower body tension
5. **ARM STRENGTH BUILDER:** build upper body power
6. **SEATED CARDIO BOOST:** get your heart pumping
7. **CORE POWER:** strengthen your center
8. **NECK AND SHOULDER RESCUE:** ease upper body tension
9. **STANDING BALANCE CHALLENGE:** improve stability (standing option)

When to Practice

- Morning: Cat-Cow Flow or Sun Salutation A to wake up
- Midday: Neck and Shoulder Rescue or Arm Strength Builder for a desk break
- Evening: Hip Mobility Magic or gentle Cat-Cow Flow to unwind
- Anytime: any sequence when you need five minutes for yourself

SEQUENCE 1: Cat–Cow Flow

Type: Gentle Spinal Warm-up and Breath-Linked Movement
Main Focus: Spine, core, neck
Secondary Focus: Shoulders, chest, hips

Perfect for: *Morning wake-up, back relief, or anytime reset*

Overview: Cat-Cow Flow is a simple yet effective spinal mobility exercise that can be done at any time to relieve tension in the back and shoulders, while gently warming up the spine and syncing breath with movement. I love to do this sequence whenever I am feeling stiff or just need a little physical reset.

Instructions:

1. Sit tall on a sturdy chair with your feet flat on the floor, hip-width apart. Rest your hands on your knees or thighs.
2. Inhale as you arch your back, lift your chest, and draw your shoulders back—gaze slightly upward for Seated Cow Pose.
3. Exhale as you round your spine, tuck your chin to your chest, and draw your belly inward into a Seated Cat Pose.
4. Continue flowing between Cow and Cat for 3–5 rounds, matching each movement with your breath.

Tip:
Sit toward the front of the chair so your spine can move freely. Keep your feet grounded and core engaged for better posture and spinal support.

Modifications:
If your feet don't comfortably touch the ground, place blocks or a folded blanket under them. For more support, keep your hands on the sides of the chair instead of your knees.

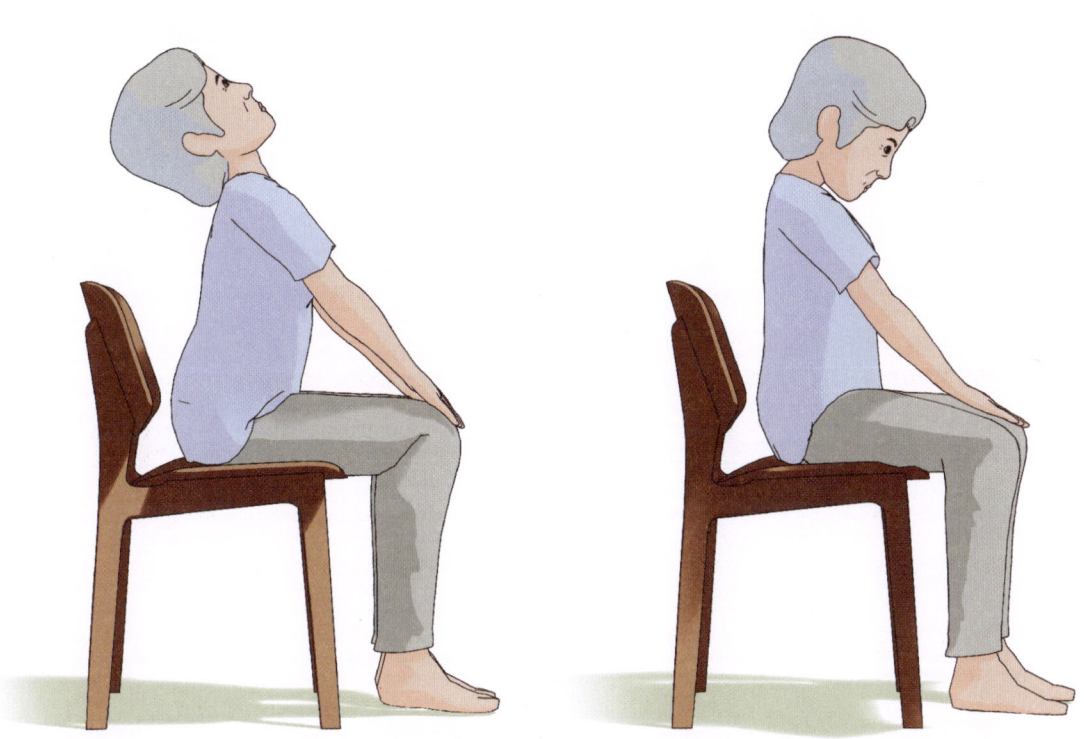

SEQUENCE 2: Sun Salutation A
(*Chair Surya Namaskar A*)

Type: Seated Flow Sequence and Full-Body Warm-up
Main Focus: Spine, shoulders, arms
Secondary Focus: Core, hips, chest

Perfect for: *Morning energy, full-body warmup, mood boost*

Overview: Chair Surya Namaskar A is an accessible adaptation of the traditional standing flow. Perfect for those with limited mobility or anyone looking to energize their body from a seated position, this sequence links breath with movement to awaken the spine, open the chest, and cultivate focus. Sun Salutation A is a ritual of movements that has been performed for decades and is very successful at moving stuck and stagnant energy.

Instructions:

1. Inhale and sweep your arms overhead, reaching toward the sky—Seated Extended Mountain Pose.
2. As you exhale, hinge at your hips and fold forward over your legs, letting your hands reach toward the floor or your shins—Seated Forward Fold.
3. Inhale and lift your chest halfway, lengthening your spine and placing your hands on your shins or thighs—Seated Half Lift.
4. Exhale and fold forward again—Seated Forward Fold.
5. Inhale and rise back up to a seated position, sweeping your arms overhead—Seated Extended Mountain Pose.
6. As you exhale, lower your hands to your heart center or rest them on your thighs—returning to Seated Equal Pose.

Tip:
Move slowly and deliberately with your breath. Sit near the front edge of your chair to allow for a fuller range of motion through your spine and hips.

Modifications:
If folding forward is uncomfortable, rest your elbows on your thighs instead of reaching toward the floor. You can also use yoga blocks or a bolster to support your hands in the forward fold.

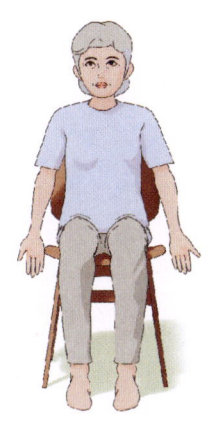

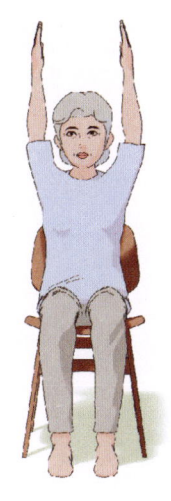

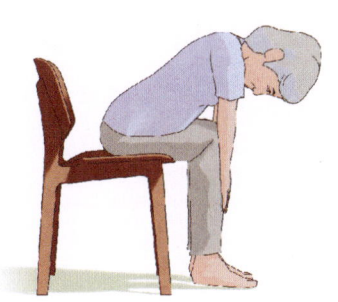

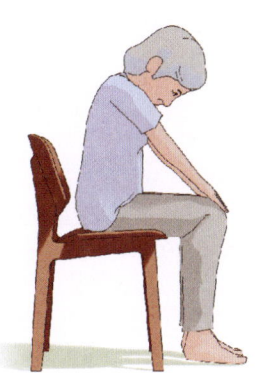

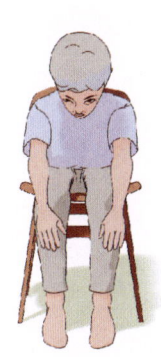

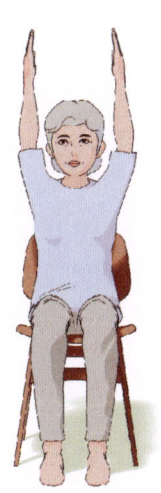

SEQUENCE 3: Sun Salutation–Warrior Flow

Type: Seated Flow Sequence, Lower Body Warm Up, Strength, and Flexibility
Main Focus: Legs, arms, torso
Secondary Focus: Hips, spine, shoulders

Perfect for: *Building heat, leg strength, confidence boost*

Overview: This seated version of the Warrior Two sequence brings strength, mobility, and grace to the body—all from your chair. It activates the legs and core, opens the hips and chest, and encourages mindful, breath-linked movement. Perfect for building stability and energy while remaining supported.

Instructions:

1. Sit facing foward on a sturdy chair, facing left with your left thigh parallel to the chair's back. Extend your right leg behind you, with your toes pointing slightly out. Keep your left knee stacked over your left ankle—Seated Warrior Two Legs.
2. Inhale and reach your left arm out in front of you and your right arm behind you, with both arms parallel to the floor. Stretch from fingertip to fingertip and gaze over your left hand—Seated Warrior Two.
3. As you exhale, lower your left forearm to your left thigh and sweep your right arm overhead, with your bicep by your ear—Seated Extended Side Angle.
4. Inhale and slide your right hand down the back of your right leg and lift your left arm up and back, creating a gentle bend—Seated Reverse Warrior.
5. Exhale and return to Seated Warrior Two. Flow through this 2–3 times.

Tip:
Keep your front knee stacked over your ankle and both feet grounded or supported. Maintain an active core and length through the spine throughout the sequence.

Modifications:
If extending your leg is difficult, keep both knees bent with feet wide and grounded.

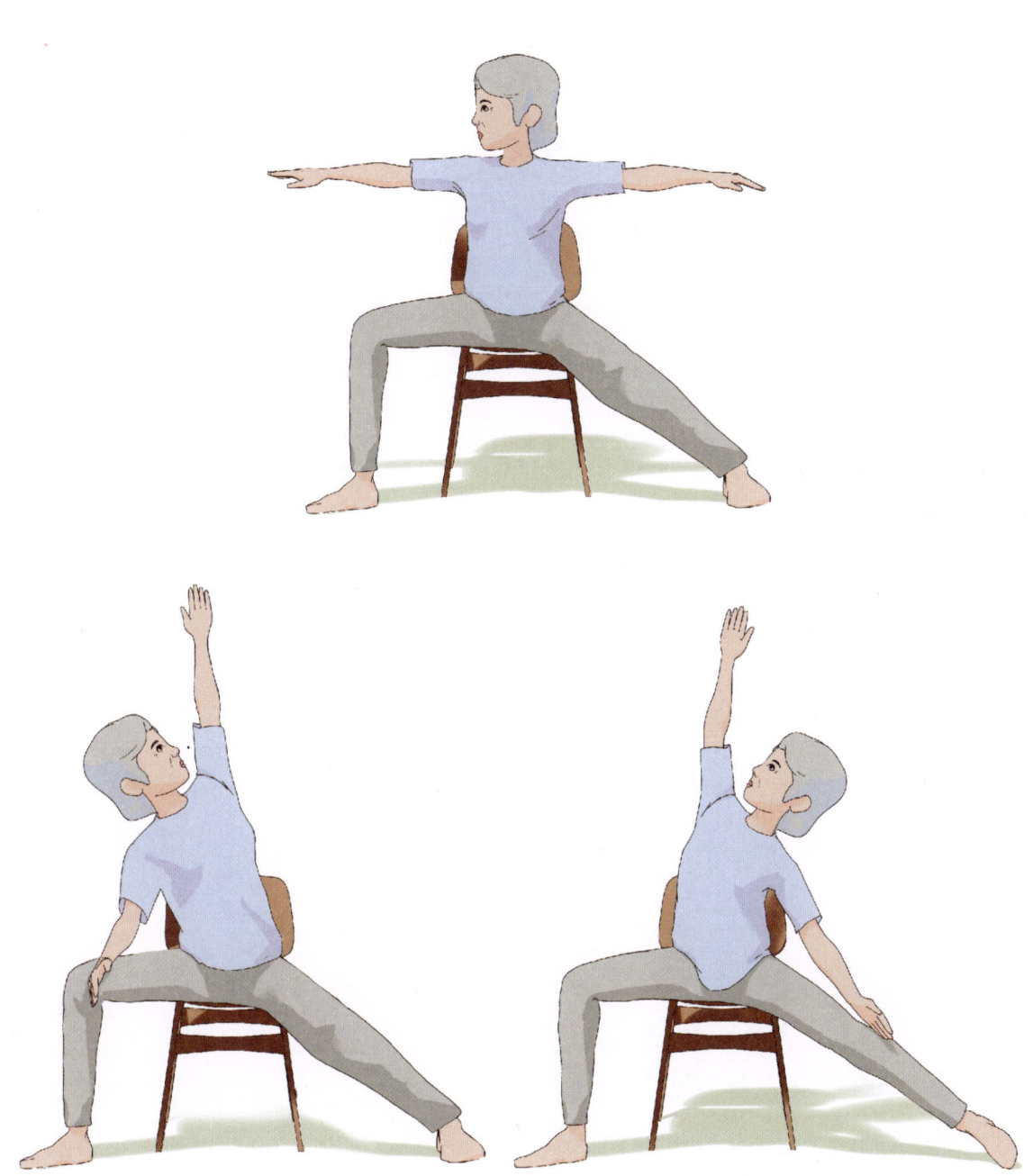

SEQUENCE 4: Hip Mobility Magic

Type: Seated Stretch and Hip Mobility Flow
Main Focus: Hips, glutes, lower back
Secondary Focus: Hamstrings, outer thighs, spine

Perfect for: *After sitting, hip tightness, lower back relief*

Overview: This seated hip mobility sequence targets deep tension in the hips, glutes, and lower back. It is ideal for people who are frequently sedentary and are looking for an increased range of motion in the lower body; the poses flow together for a well-rounded hip release.

Instructions:

1. Inhale and draw your left knee toward your chest, clasping it gently with both hands. Sit up tall and lengthen through your spine as you hug your knee in. Hold for 3–5 breaths—Seated Half Wind Removing Pose.
2. Exhale and cross your left ankle over your right thigh, flexing your left foot. Sit up tall and gently press your left knee downward to open the hip. Hold for several breaths—Seated Figure Four.
3. Next, cross your left leg fully over your right (stacking knees if possible). Inhale to sit tall, then exhale to fold forward, letting your hands rest on your thighs, your shins, or the floor. Breathe deeply into the outer hips and back body—Shoelace Pose with a Fold.
4. Inhale as you raise your upper body, uncross your legs, and return to a neutral seated position. Repeat the full sequence on your left side.

Tip:
Keep both feet flexed during any cross-legged shapes to protect your knees.

Modifications:
Perform a gentler figure four by keeping your ankle on your thigh and skipping the full shoelace. Place yoga blocks or a folded blanket under your feet if they don't reach the floor.

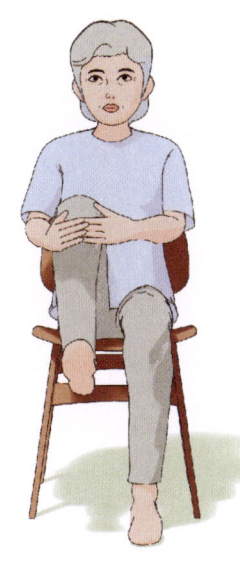

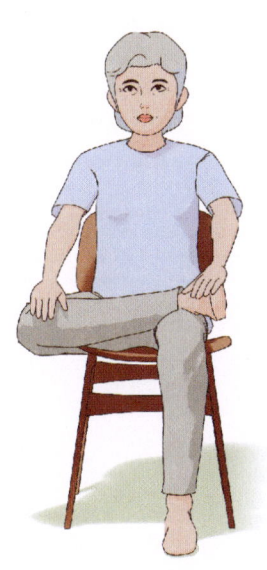

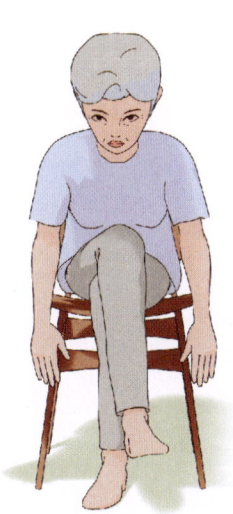

SEQUENCE NUMBER 5: Arm Strength Builder

Type: Seated Strength-Building Flow
Main Focus: Arms, shoulders, wrists
Secondary Focus: Upper back, posture

Perfect for: *Desk break, building strength, improving posture*

Overview: This seated sequence is designed to build strength and endurance in your arms and shoulders while improving mobility in your wrists. Perfect for those who spend time typing or doing repetitive hand and arm movements, these simple exercises can be done with or without weights and offer a great way to tone and support the upper body.

Instructions:

1. Extend your arms forward at shoulder height, palms facing down. Inhale to flex your wrists (fingers pointing up), then exhale to point them down. Repeat for 6–8 rounds, moving with your breath—Arm Raise with Flex and Point.
2. Raise both arms and keep elbows close to your sides, arms bent at 90 degrees. Inhale to lower your forearms, then exhale to curl them up toward your shoulders. Continue for 8–12 slow reps. Add light weights or resistance bands for a challenge—Seated Yogi Bicep Curls.
3. Inhale, reach both arms forward at shoulder height with your palms down. Then exhale, open your arms out to a T shape. Inhale and bring them back to the center. Repeat for 6–10 rounds, moving slowly and with control—Forward to T Arm Extensions—Seated Double Arm Frontal Raise to T Arms.
4. Extend your arms out to the sides at shoulder height. Make small circles forward for 10–15 seconds, then reverse. Keep your shoulders relaxed and your core gently engaged—Micro Arm Circles.

Tip:
Focus on slow, controlled movements to get the most benefit. Keep your neck and jaw relaxed, and sit tall with your feet grounded.

Modifications:
Lower your arms at any time to reduce the range of motion. Or perform the sequence one arm at a time for added support.

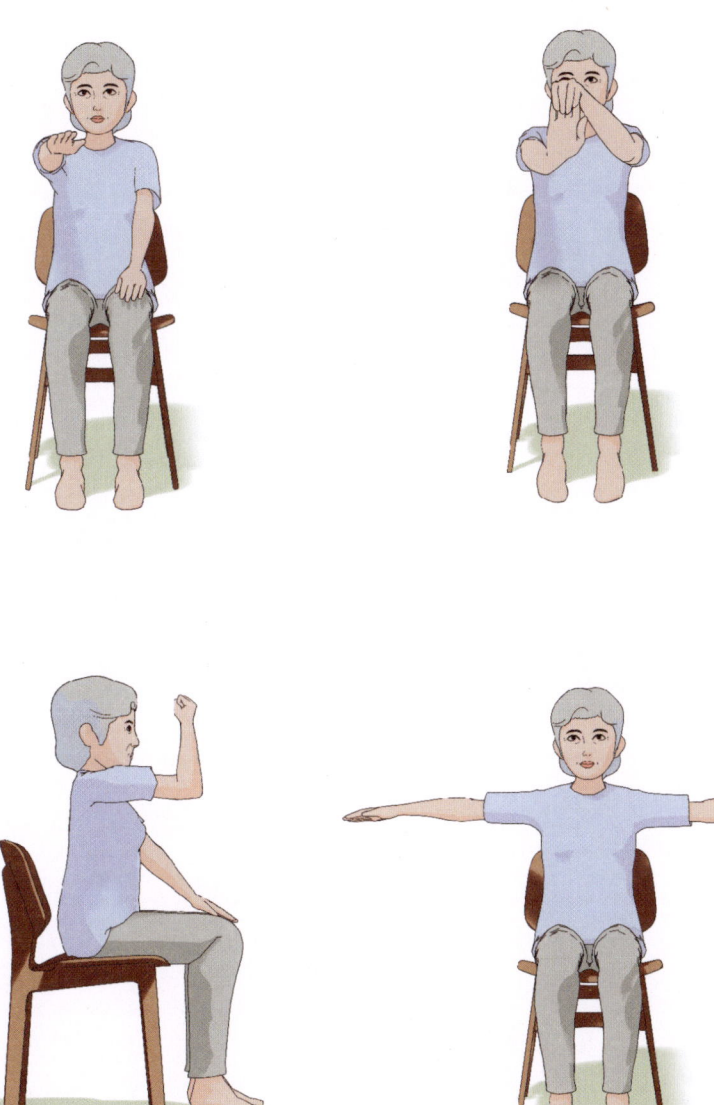

SEQUENCE 6: Seated Cardio Boost

Type: Low-Impact Cardio
Main Focus: Legs, arms, core, cardiovascular system
Secondary Focus: Heart, shoulders, coordination

Perfect for: *Afternoon slump, gentle cardio, improving circulation*

Overview: This seated cardio sequence is designed to gently elevate the heart rate while staying grounded in your chair. Through rhythmic leg and arm lifts, you'll build circulation, coordination, and light strength. Perfect as a warm-up or a quick pick-me-up at any time during the day.

Instructions:

1. Sit tall with your feet flat on the floor. Inhale and lift your left knee toward your chest. Exhale and lower it down. Inhale and lift your right knee. Exhale and lower it. Continue alternating for 30–60 seconds—Seated Marching Legs.
2. Inhale as you sweep both arms up overhead. Exhale and lower them down to your sides. Repeat for 5–8 rounds, linking movement with breath—Arm Raises with Breath.
3. Inhale and lift your right arm and left leg at the same time. Exhale and lower them. Inhale and lift your left arm and right leg. Exhale as you lower them. Continue alternating for 6–10 slow reps per side—Opposite Arm and Leg Lifts.

Tip:
Move at your own pace and keep your breath steady. Engage your core and sit tall at the edge of your chair for better posture and support.

Modifications:
If needed, lift only the arms or legs instead of both together. Add light hand or ankle weights to increase the intensity when you're ready.

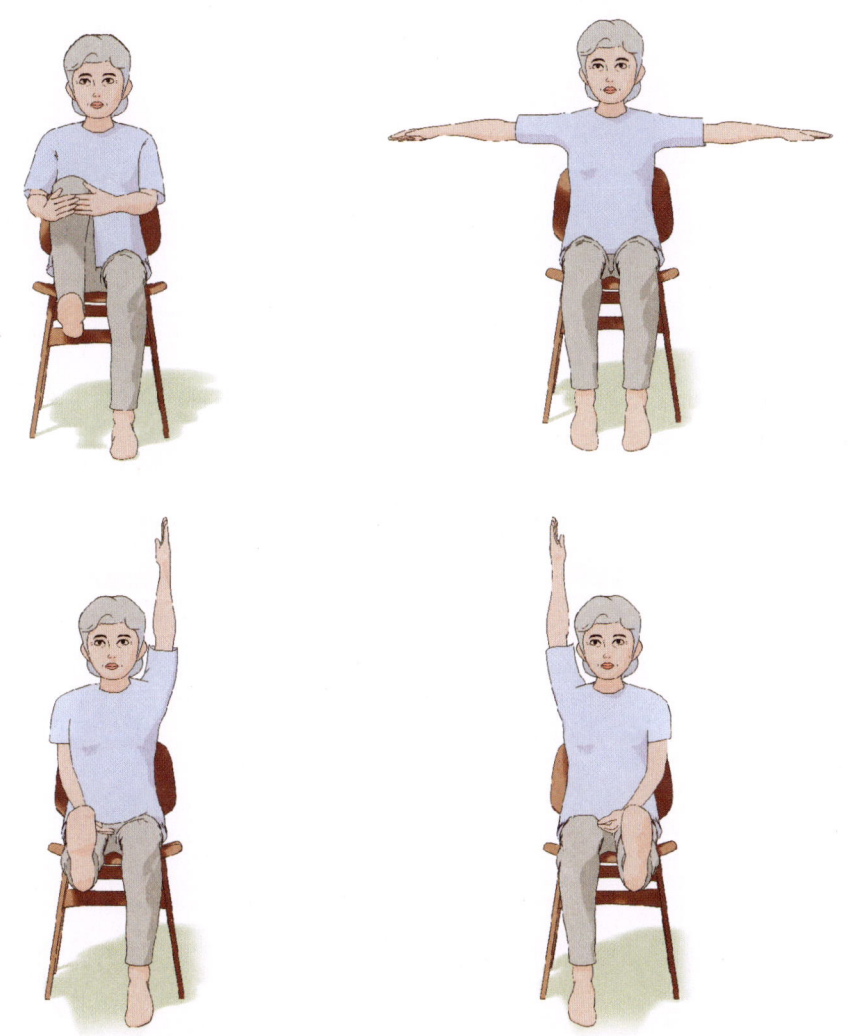

SEQUENCE 7: Core Power

Type: Core Strengthening
Main Focus: Abdominals, obliques, spine
Secondary Focus: Posture, breath awareness, deep core engagement

Perfect for: *Core strength, improved posture, spinal support*

Overview: This seated core sequence is designed to activate and strengthen your abdominal muscles. With intentional crunching movements and mindful breath, you'll tone your midsection, support your spine, and build a solid foundation of strength. Great as a stand-alone series or as part of a full-body seated routine.

Instructions:

1. Sit tall near the edge of your chair, with your feet flat and hip-width apart. Interlace your hands behind your head with your elbows wide. Inhale to prepare. Exhale, engage your core, and gently round your upper spine as you bring your ribs toward your hips. Inhale, returning to a tall spine. Repeat for 5–8 reps—Seated Crunches.
2. From the same seated position, keep your hands behind your head. Inhale to lengthen. Exhale, then rotate and crunch your torso as you bring your right elbow toward your left knee (lift the knee if comfortable). Inhale as you move back to the center. Exhale and bring your left elbow to your right knee. Continue alternating for 4–8 reps per side—Oblique Crunches.

Tip:
Focus on small, controlled movements. Keep your core engaged throughout and avoid pulling on your neck. Slow and steady wins the core game.

Modifications:
Keep both feet on the floor and focus just on the torso rotation if lifting the knees is too difficult. To increase intensity, hold the crunch briefly at the top of each rep.

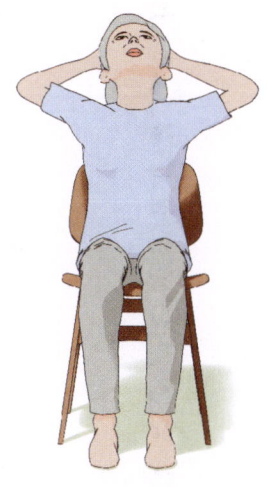

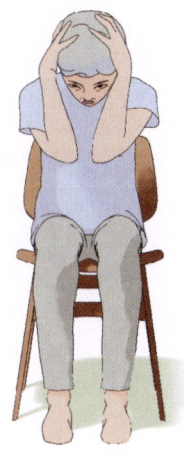

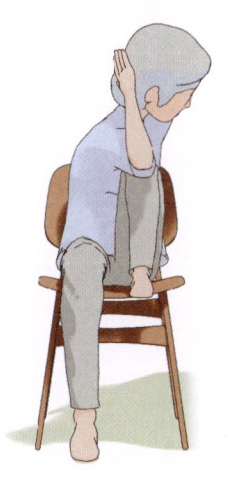

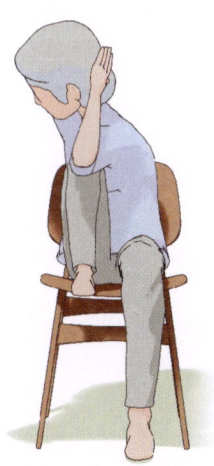

01 14

SEQUENCE 8: Neck and Shoulder Rescue

Type: Gentle Stretch and Mobility
Main Focus: Neck, shoulders
Secondary Focus: Jaw, upper spine, nervous system

Perfect for: *Computer work breaks, tension headaches, stress relief*

Overview: This calming neck release sequence is perfect for easing tension in the upper body. Ideal after screen time or as a grounding pause during your day, these simple moves help restore mobility and relaxation. I love to do this when I'm feeling tense or first thing in the morning when I wake up!

Instructions:

1. Sit tall. Drop your right ear toward your right shoulder. Inhale back to the center. Exhale and drop your left ear to your left shoulder. Repeat 3–5 rounds per side—Seated Ear to Shoulder Pose.
2. Drop your chin to your chest. Inhale and gently tilt your head back. Inhale as you move back to the center. Repeat 3–5 times—Chin to Chest Pose with Tilts.
3. Turn your head to the right. Inhale as you return to the center. Turn your head to the left, then back to the center. Repeat for 3–5 rounds—Neck Twists.
4. Drop your chin and slowly circle your head in one direction, then the other. Repeat the movement 2–3 times each way—Neck Rolls.
5. Inhale as you lift your shoulders upward, then exhale and drop them back and down. Roll your shoulders backward and forward for 5–8 rounds each—Shoulder Rolls.

Tip:
Move slowly, breathe steadily, and relax your jaw.

Modifications:
Skip full neck rolls if they feel too intense. Use a backrest for support if needed.

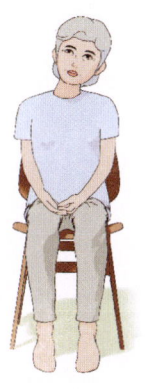
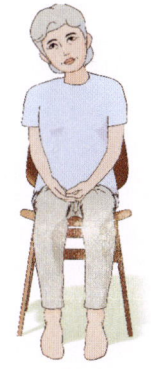
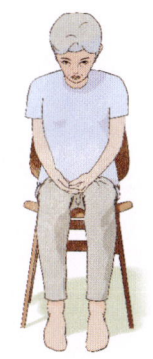

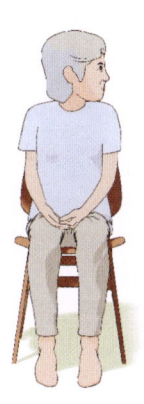
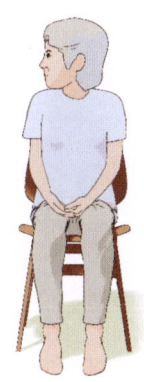
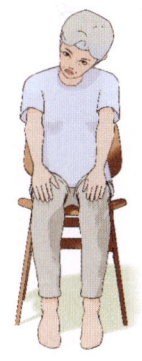

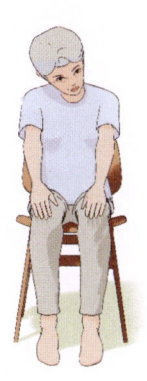
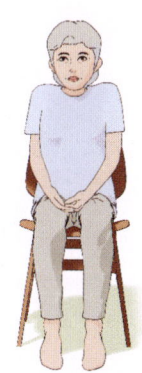
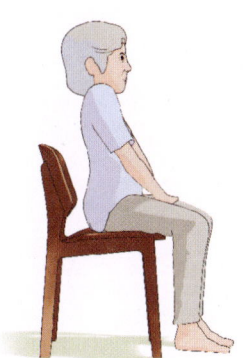
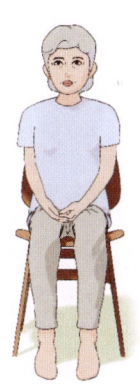

SEQUENCE 9: Standing Balance Challenge

Type: Supported Standing Series
Main Focus: Legs, hips, core, balance
Secondary Focus: Posture, ankle stability, confidence, proprioception

Perfect for: *Building confidence, improving balance, leg strength*

Overview: This series builds lower-body strength and balance using a chair for support. You'll challenge your stability while staying safe and supported.

Disclaimer: These are more advanced postures and should only be practiced if you can comfortably stand steadily without additional support.

Instructions:

1. Stand behind your chair, with your hands on the backrest and your feet hip-width apart. Inhale, bend your knees, and lower into a gentle squat. Exhale and press into your feet to rise. Repeat for 5–8 reps—Chair Squats.
2. Stand tall with your hands on the back of the chair. Inhale and lift your left knee to hip height. Exhale and lower it. Switch sides. Continue alternating for 4–6 lifts per side—Knee Lifts.
3. Stand tall with one hand on the back of the chair. Place your left foot on the inside of your right ankle or shin. Press your foot gently into the leg. Hold for 3–5 breaths. Switch sides—Supported Tree Pose.
4. Facing the back of the chair, step your right foot back with your toes angled out. Bend your left knee. Place both hands on the chair for support, and keep your spine long. Hold for 3–5 breaths, then switch sides—Supported Standing Warrior One.
5. Stand sideways to the chair, with one hand resting on the back of the chair. Take a large step back with your right foot, keeping your left toes facing forward and your right toes turned slightly out.
6. Bend your left knee, and extend the other arm out. Hold for 3–5 breaths, then switch sides—Supported Standing Warrior Two.

Tip:
Keep a soft bend in the standing knee, and engage your core. Use the chair for support, not as a crutch—build trust in your body.

Modifications:
Keep your movements smaller or hold onto the chair with both hands if needed.

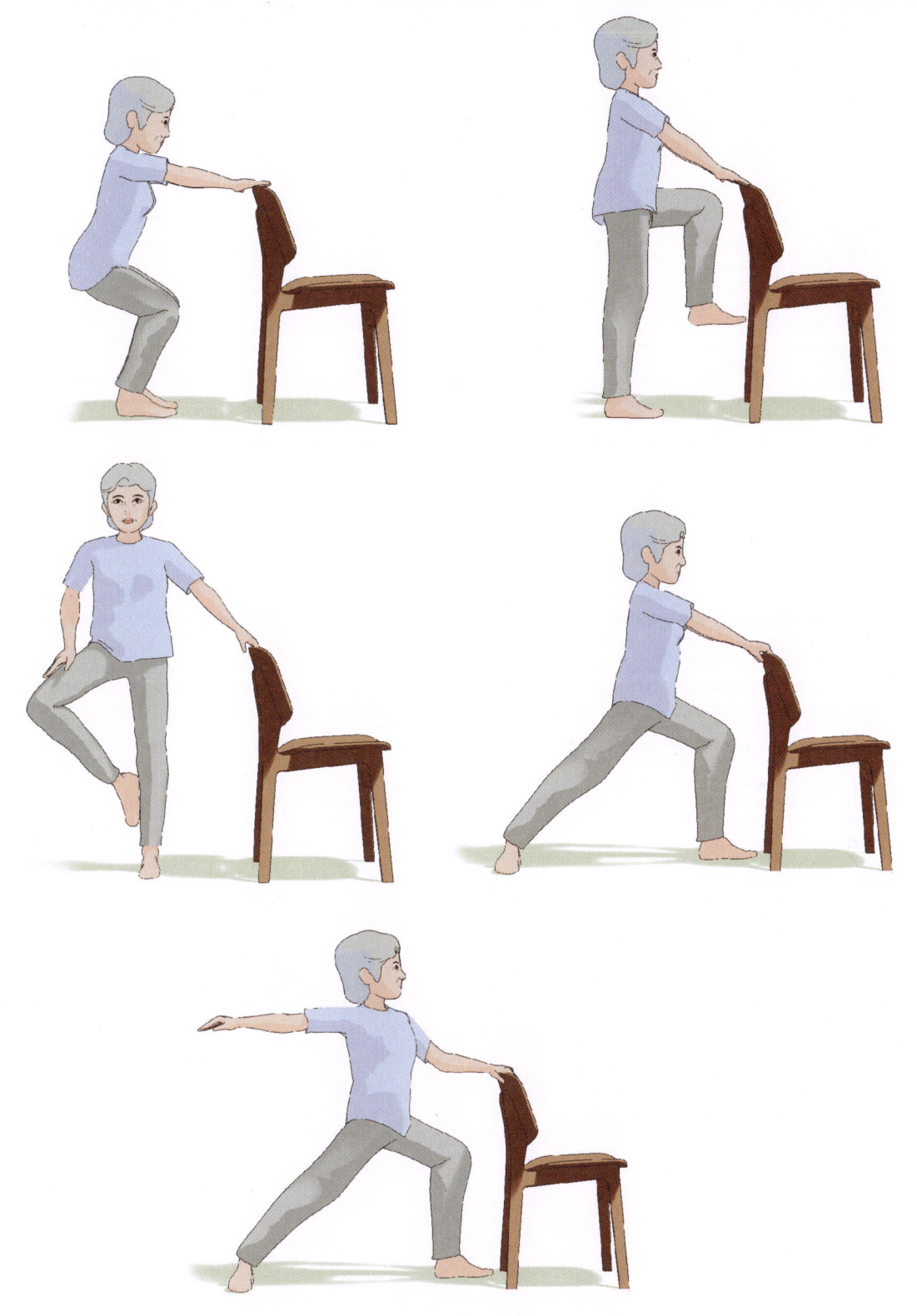

CREATE YOUR PERFECT DAY

Sample Daily 5-Minute Plan

- 7 a.m.: Sun Salutation A (wake up)
- 12 p.m.: Neck and Shoulder Rescue (lunch break)
- 5 p.m.: Hip Mobility Magic (after work)

6 a.m.	6 p.m.
7 a.m.	7 p.m.
8 a.m.	8 p.m.
9 a.m.	9 p.m.
10 a.m.	10 p.m.
11 a.m.	11 p.m.
12 p.m.	12 a.m.
1 p.m.	1 a.m.
2 p.m.	2 a.m.
3 p.m.	3 a.m.
4 p.m.	4 a.m.
5 p.m.	5 a.m.

Weekly Practice Ideas

- Monday/Wednesday/Friday: Strength focus (Arms, Core, Balance)
- Tuesday/Thursday: Flexibility focus (Cat-Cow, Hip Mobility, Neck)
- Weekend: Your choice—what does your body need?

MONDAY	
TUESDAY	
WEDNESDAY	
THURSDAY	
FRIDAY	
SATURDAY	
SUNDAY	

Conclusion

Congratulations on completing this chair yoga journey! You've taken important steps toward improving your flexibility, strength, and overall well-being. By practicing these poses and sequences, you've already started to experience the benefits of mindful movement and body awareness.

Remember the key to continuing your progress is consistency. Incorporate what you've learned here into your daily routine, whether it's a quick stretch in the morning or a full session when you need to unwind. Don't hesitate to explore new variations or modify the movements to suit your needs.

Yoga is a lifelong practice—one that adapts with you as you grow stronger and more confident. Continue to listen to your body, be patient, and practice with intention. The mat, or in this case, the chair, is always there when you're ready to continue your journey.

You've proven you can do this. Your chair is waiting for you when you need it, and our 5-minute practice is always available. And remember it's never too late to begin again; to create a loving relationship with yourself, your body, and your mind.

Keep this book handy. Return to it often. Let these 5-minute practices become anchors in your day—moments of movement, breath, and self-care that remind you of your strength and resilience.

With love and admiration for your journey,
Kierstie

Acknowledgments

With deep gratitude, thank you to the incredible seniors I've had the honor of teaching. Watching you all show up with curiosity, courage, and grace has been one of the greatest inspirations of my life. Your willingness to embrace yoga later in life is a powerful reminder that it's never too late to grow, heal, and connect more deeply with ourselves. You've shown me how transformative this practice can be—physically, mentally, and spiritually.

To all the teachers who came before me, thank you for passing down the wisdom and heart of yoga. To my family and friends, your love and constant encouragement have been my foundation. And to Sasquatch Books, thank you for believing in this project and giving me the nudge to share this work with a wider community.

This book is for all of you—it exists because of you.

Index

S

About the Author

KIERSTIE PAYGE DOLEZAL is an international yoga educator, retreat leader, and experienced 500-hour yoga teacher (500 E-RYT) known for her bold, heart-centered approach to the practice. With thousands of hours of teaching and training experience, she blends her athletic roots with deep studies in yogic philosophy, bringing a rich and grounded perspective to her leadership.

Kierstie has guided students across the globe—offering training, workshops, and retreats that challenge, inspire, and awaken. She's passionate about making yoga accessible to all, and over the past eight years, has developed a powerful connection to the senior community. From memory care centers to online classes viewed by millions, she's witnessed firsthand how yoga can reignite joy, spark healing, and transform lives—at any age.

Her teaching honors ancient traditions while inviting students to explore their edge with curiosity and compassion. Whether in a studio, a care facility, or on retreat, Kierstie reminds us that freedom is not found, but remembered—a truth buried deep within. Yoga is the ancient map that leads you back to yourself, breath by breath, layer by layer.